MINDFULNESS AND THE THERAPEUTIC RELATIONSHIP

MINDFULNESS and the THERAPEUTIC RELATIONSHIP

Edited by
STEVEN F. HICK
THOMAS BIEN

Foreword by Zindel V. Segal

THE GUILFORD PRESS
New York   London

Printed in the United States of America

This book is printed on acid-free paper.

Last digit is print number: 9   8   7   6   5   4   3   2   1

Library of Congress Cataloging-in-Publication Data

Hick, Steven F.
  Mindfulness and the therapeutic relationship / edited by Steven F. Hick, Thomas
Bien.
       p. ; cm.
  Includes bibliographical references and index.
  ISBN 978-1-59385-820-9 (hardcover : alk. paper)
  1. Psychotherapist and patient.   2. Meditation—Therapeutic use.   3. Attention.
4. Awareness.   I. Bien, Thomas.   II. Title.
  [DNLM: 1. Meditation—methods.   2. Psychotherapy—methods.   3. Awareness.
4. Meditation—psychology.   5. Professional–Patient Relations.
  WM 425.5.R3 H627m 2008]
  RC489.M43H53 2008
  616.89′14—dc22

                                                                        2008010080

About the Editors

Steven F. Hick, PhD, RSW, is Associate Professor in the School of Social Work at Carleton University in Ottawa, Ontario, Canada, where he teaches in the areas of mindfulness, human rights practice, social worker formation, and community development. The author or editor of a number of books, including the leading social work text in Canada, Dr. Hick is at the forefront in the use of mindfulness in social work practice, and has recently begun research on mindfulness. He is co-founder of War Child Canada, a nonprofit organization that helps children affected by war.

Thomas Bien, PhD, is a psychologist in private practice in Albuquerque, New Mexico, where he teaches mindfulness and meditation. The author or coauthor of several books on mindfulness, Dr. Bien conducts national and international presentations, and has played an influential role in integrating mindfulness into the practice of psychotherapy.

Contributors

Thomas Bien, PhD, private practice, Albuquerque, New Mexico

Sarah Bowen, PhD, Addictive Behaviors Research Center, Department of Psychology, University of Washington, Seattle, Washington

Neha Chawla, MS, Addictive Behaviors Research Center, Department of Psychology, University of Washington, Seattle, Washington

Paul R. Fulton, EdD, Tufts Health Plan, Newton Center, Massachusetts

Diane Gehart, PhD, LMFT, Department of Educational Psychology and Counseling, California State University, Northridge, Northridge, California

Steven F. Hick, PhD, School of Social Work, Carleton University, Ottawa, Ontario, Canada

Christin D. Izett, MA, Department of Psychology, Santa Clara University, Santa Clara, California

Gregory Kramer, PhD, Metta Foundation, Portland, Oregon

Michael J. Lambert, PhD, Department of Psychology, Brigham Young University, Provo, Utah

Mishka Lysack, PhD, Faculty of Social Work, University of Calgary, and Calgary Family Therapy Centre, Calgary, Alberta, Canada

G. Alan Marlatt, PhD, Addictive Behaviors Research Center, Department of Psychology, University of Washington, Seattle, Washington

Eric E. McCollum, PhD, LCSW, LMFT, Marriage and Family Therapy Program, Virginia Tech University–Northern Virginia Center, Falls Church, Virginia

Florence Meleo-Meyer, MA, Center for Mindfulness, University of Massachusetts Medical School, Worcester, Massachusetts

Romy Reading, MA, Department of Psychology, New School for Social Research, New York, New York

Jeremy D. Safran, PhD, Department of Psychology, New School for Social Research, New York, New York

Emily K. Sandoz, MS, Department of Psychology, University of Mississippi, University, Mississippi

Rebecca Shafir, MA, CCC, Hallowell Center for Cognitive and Emotional Health, Sudbury, Massachusetts

Shauna L. Shapiro, PhD, Department of Counseling Psychology, Santa Clara University, Santa Clara, California

Witold Simon, MD, PhD, Department of Neurotic Disorders and Psychotherapy, Institute of Psychiatry and Neurology, Warsaw, Poland

Martha Lee Turner, PhD, Metta Foundation, Evanston, Illinois

Russell A. Walsh, PhD, Psychology Department, Duquesne University, Pittsburgh, Pennsylvania

Kelly G. Wilson, PhD, Psychology Department, University of Mississippi, University, Mississippi

Katie Witkiewitz, PhD, Alcohol and Drug Abuse Institute, Department of Psychology, University of Washington, Seattle, Washington

Foreword

These are interesting times in which to be a psychotherapist. We are witnessing one of the signal events of the new millennium in our field, namely, the intersection of two previously separate approaches to human suffering. One tradition dates back 2,500 years and teaches a calm abiding amidst insistent mental activity, whereas the other, while existing unformed for many years, was formally structured over the last century and brings analysis and narrative to bear on mental states and symptoms. Mindfulness and psychotherapy have quite naturally found each other in ways that allow both patients and therapists to reap the benefits of embedding awareness practices within a traditional therapeutic frame. In this important volume, Steven Hick, Thomas Bien, and their contributors embark on a much-needed discussion of the contours of this emerging synthesis, through a multifaceted examination of the connection between the therapeutic relationship and mindfulness practice.

The scope of the chapters and range of topics covered, in both the clinical adaptations of mindfulness and empirical findings on the therapeutic alliance, are comprehensive. There is also considerable clarity, wisdom, and restraint in the discussion of how much we know and still do not know about this young union—qualities that are often lacking in the wake of this area's burgeoning growth. This book is also home to a number of polar constructs that seem to require resolution in binary terms, especially concerning distressed patients or requests to teach others about mindfulness-based clinical care. Are we imparting skills or presence? Is this therapy or personal growth? Are we encouraging problem solving or subjective unfolding? The literature on the therapeutic relationship and writings on mindfulness can offer some answers, but the beauty of this book is that it allows the reader to look at the space between these two sources and see how a bridge between them, perhaps a trestle at first, is starting to be built.

ZINDEL V. SEGAL, PHD
Centre for Addiction and Mental Health
University of Toronto

Preface

The work of the busy therapist is full of struggles with third-party payers, scheduling, answering phone calls, creating and maintaining accurate records, establishing treatment plans, meeting the requirements of licensing boards, and many other activities peripheral to the work of therapy. At times it may seem as though meetings with clients were the interruption, while these other matters were primary. While it is easy to get caught in this trap on occasion, therapists know that their clients are what really matter. Being fully present for them requires that a therapist be able to put other matters aside and become deeply quiet, open, and receptive. The capacity to do so is the *sine qua non* of a healing therapeutic relationship. Another name for this capacity is mindfulness.

The initial idea for this book came from my (SFH) gradual realization that it was relationship and not technique that underlies all successful interventions, be it in an individual, group, or community setting. Furthermore, I found that by teaching relationship skills in community organizations, amazing things began to happen. Increasingly, people began to respond to one another with compassion, understanding, and deep appreciation. Similar events transpired in my group work. With groups, I prepare to be mindful on two levels, not only scheduling the activities carefully, but also attempting to bring a sense of calm and inner peace to myself before sessions. Repeatedly, I found if I missed the first preparation I could still improvise and the class would evolve without difficulty. But if I was not mindfully prepared, things inevitably went astray. Books on delivering mindfulness programs all make this point, but I found little specific discussion of the issues and practice.

I (TB), on the other hand, was concurrently discovering the same truth in the context of my work as a therapist. When I was calm and centered, doors seemed to open in therapy that would have remained closed were I distracted, preoccupied, or even just overanxious to be helpful. Yet when I read the growing literature on mindfulness-based interventions, they seemed to emphasize technique over relationship. These ongoing reflections eventually became embodied in my *Mindful Therapy* book, with which I hoped to begin to fill this gap.

In the light of our experience of the value of the relationship, recent calls for empirically validated treatments predicated upon specific treatment models seemed somewhat suspect. Surprisingly little variance in outcome is actually due to this factor. Instead, the *quality* of the therapeutic relationship has consistently correlated more highly with client outcome than specialized therapy *techniques* (see, for example, Chapter 2, this volume).

While specific techniques can be helpful, we each continued to experience that presence, deep listening, compassion, and a sense of interconnection were the most important determinants of outcome. And indeed, some preliminary findings from a few studies (see Chapter 1 for a review of these) support the anecdotal evidence. It may even be the case that technique is important because it facilitates the therapeutic relationship—perhaps through the installation of a sense of hope—rather than relationship being important because it supports technique.

One of the editors (TB) recently attended a conference regarding the cognitive-behavioral treatment of anxiety disorders. When the presenter offhandedly expressed a bias against mindfulness approaches, a participant agreed, remarking that psychology is periodically embarrassed by faddish and fleeting movements of this kind.

If mindfulness is a fad, it is one that has survived for over 25 centuries. If it has not been tested until recently, through controlled clinical trials, it has nonetheless stood the test of time, largely through the tradition of Buddhist teaching. Since that tradition has a profoundly empirical, experiential attitude, it is not so surprising that it is attractive to the modern, scientifically trained therapist. The traditional mindfulness practices known today have been passed on from generation to generation, refined by the fires of time and experience, and by their introduction into diverse lingual and cultural contexts.

Indeed, from this perspective one could argue that psychology, as we think of it, is the upstart, and mindfulness the established empirical method—if we understand empirical in the broad sense of being based on reliable and repeatable experience rather than a narrowly scientific emphasis on controlled clinical trials. Given the longstanding track record of mindfulness, testing whether mindfulness helps may not be the most interesting question to ask. As mindfulness is accepted into clinical experience and research, other questions emerge: *How* does mindfulness help? For what conditions and disorders? How is it best taught to clients? What sorts of exercises are most beneficial? And, as Buddhist practitioners have asked through the ages, how is it best approached in this time, in these places, within the current cultural contexts?

Perhaps even more important questions than these, however, are ones that have scarcely been asked until now. For example, what kind of effect does the practice of mindfulness by a therapist, counselor, or community worker have on the therapeutic relationship and the outcome? How can mindfulness be taught to helping professionals? How can those who already practice mindfulness bring that practice into the therapy room or their community work? In this volume, we hope to begin addressing these issues.

In Part I we explore the terrain of mindfulness and the therapeutic relationship, defining and uncovering key issues and examining existing research and literature. Part II takes us further into key aspects of the therapeutic relationship within a mindfulness approach. Difficult concepts such as compassion, non-self, and empathy are discussed and disentangled. Part III takes up these issues within the context of specific treatment approaches. Here we see how mindfulness can contribute to positive therapeutic relationships within specific interventions. Bringing this all together, Part IV provides some advice and lessons learned from actual experience in teaching and learning mindfulness for cultivating positive relationships.

Acknowledgments

In preparing this book I (SFH) have been helped by many friends. I am deeply grateful to all of my students for their support and insightful questions and reflections. I would be remiss without thanking my wife, Vaida, and my children, Kristina and Justin, for being supportive as I wandered off on yet another 7-day or 10-day mindfulness retreat. While it is not common for coeditors to express appreciation for one another, I feel that it is absolutely necessary in this case. I suffered a concussion and lost my ability for advanced thinking in the midst of the editing process, and Thomas Bien was unflappable and kind in picking up the many pieces that I let fall through the cracks.

I (TB) thank my many teachers in psychology, and the many spiritual teachers—Christian, Jewish, Hindu, and Buddhist—I encountered along the way. They are far too numerous to try to mention. Regarding spiritual teachers, I especially acknowledge Thich Nhat Hanh, whose books continue to instruct and inspire me in the art of mindful living, and whose presence on retreat has provided an example of living Buddhahood. I deeply appreciate Steven Hick's invitation to join him in this project. I am also grateful for the work of our contributors through sometimes difficult revisions. None of us works in a bubble, but must do our best through the difficulties of living, and this applies to everyone involved in this book as well. Some of these difficulties have been known to us; undoubtedly many others have not. I am grateful for my clients and students, most of whom, thankfully, have been kind and appreciative teachers, some of whom have been more difficult though also helpful. Finally, I am always deeply grateful for my wife, Beverly, and her kind presence in my life.

Contents

I THEORY AND PRACTICE

What is mindfulness? What does mindfulness have to do with the practice of psychotherapy? In this section, we consider what mindfulness is, and what its true importance may be in the practice of psychotherapy.

Steven Hick takes us through the conceptual issues of defining mindfulness, considering mindfulness in its dual aspect of both a technique and a way of facilitating therapeutic presence. He describes currently available methods for measuring mindfulness, and considers the problem of the objective measurement of such a subjective experience. He reviews five studies showing that mindfulness can have a positive impact on the therapeutic relationship.

Michael Lambert and Witold Simon clarify the issues of concept definition and measurement of the therapeutic relationship. Partitioning of the variance in psychotherapy outcome research reveals that relationship factors are more important than specific clinical technique. Yet there are difficulties in providing training in the sort of empathic attitude associated with positive outcome. They offer an empirically supported device for tracking the therapeutic relationship.

1 Cultivating Therapeutic Relationships

The Role of Mindfulness

Steven F. Hick

This chapter introduces what mindfulness is, how it is cultivated, and why it is important to the relationship between clients and therapists, group counselors, community workers, and other mental health professionals. The more in-depth discussion and overview of empirical research on how the therapeutic relationship is vital in contributing to client progress and clinical outcome is reserved for Chapter 2. This book is necessary for two primary reasons. First, as Chapter 2 indicates, the therapeutic relationship is crucial for effective therapy or group work. In fact, some clinicians have found that it is more important than the type of intervention that is followed. Second, mindfulness has the potential to play a central role in enhancing the therapeutic relationship.

Defining mindfulness is a paradoxical undertaking, especially if one intends to use just words. For one thing, mindfulness really must be experienced to be understood. Further, mindfulness can be considered a preconceptual and presymbolic notion. It is an embodied state of being that cannot be accurately described using language. I have found that as my mindfulness practice develops, word-based definitions seem to capture less and less of its essence. Having said this, one must note that numerous researchers have delved into defining mindfulness and in the process have helped clarify and concretize it, especially, perhaps, for people that do not practice it. It is defined by some as having a spiritual quality and by others within a strictly scientific orientation. Still others combine the two, seeking scientific evidence for what are essentially traditional spiritual practices. Most see it as a way of living or being in the world, rather than a set of techniques—a path that is cultivated through experience rather than absorbed from a book. So, while the theory in this book may be helpful in formulating mindfulness and its uses for the therapeutic relationship, ultimately you may need to "sit quietly and breathe" and perhaps engage some of the exercises contained in the book.

Practitioners such as psychotherapists, social workers, psychiatrists, family therapists, and other mental health professionals, as well as medical doctors, are showing extraordinary interest in mindfulness as it affects practice, both for themselves and their clients. There is unparalleled interest in mindfulness-based interventions and approaches for a range of issues such as addictions, suicide, depression, trauma, and HIV/AIDS, to name a few. As the chapters in this book indicate, there is mounting interest in mindfulness practice as training through which the professional can cultivate empathy and compassion or develop a sense of presence or listening skills. Mindfulness can have an impact on how practitioners relate to their clients. This is often referred to as the therapeutic relationship (for an in-depth examination of the therapeutic relationship see Chapter 2). Beyond directly affecting client–therapist interaction, mindfulness can alter how practitioners cope with stressful events in their lives both at work and at home. Because of this, many employers of mental health professionals see mindfulness as a potential means for reducing worker turnover or so-called burnout (Wheat, 2005).

Anecdotal evidence from delivering a mindfulness-based group intervention called radical mindfulness training (an adapted version of mindfulness-based stress reduction [MBSR]) leads me to conclude that a key ingredient for positive outcome lies in the relationship that develops between the facilitator and the clients, or what we are calling the therapeutic relationship in this book. The research that is examined in this book highlights the centrality of the therapeutic relationship as a primary factor contributing to positive client outcome. When it comes to exploring how mindfulness might contribute to the therapeutic relationship, there is a gap in the existing literature—a gap this book aims to address.

MINDFULNESS IN A THERAPEUTIC CONTEXT

Mindfulness has been described as focusing attention, being aware, intentionality, being nonjudgmental, acceptance, and compassion. Mark Lau and his team at the Centre for Addiction and Mental Health in Toronto collated definitions from Kabat-Zinn (1990), Shapiro, Schwartz, and Bonner (1998), and Segal, Williams, and Teasdale (2002), who describe mindfulness as a nonelaborative, nonjudgmental, present-centered awareness in which each thought, feeling, or sensation that arises in the attentional field is acknowledged and accepted as it is. The present-centered awareness or way of paying attention is cultivated, sustained, and integrated into everything that one does, including one's therapy or community work. At the base of mindfulness is an ongoing meditation practice or other exercises that propel deep inquiry. Many elements contained within mindfulness can be traced back to centuries-old meditative traditions.

Within the client–therapist relationship, mindfulness is a way of paying attention with empathy, presence, and deep listening that can be cultivated, sustained, and integrated into our work as therapists through the ongoing discipline of meditation practice. Mindfulness can be thought of as a kind of shift from a "doing mode" to a "being mode." We tend to spend much of our time as "human doings," running from one activity to another—living our lives as though on a perpetual treadmill. This way of living distracts us from our lives. The being mode places the therapist directly in the here-and-now encounter with the client. Mindfulness meditation is an example of an activity that exemplifies the being mode. It is a nonjudgmental moment-to-moment awareness.

Larry Rosenberg (1998, p. 15), a meditation teacher, likens mindfulness to a mirror simply reflecting what is there. He emphasizes the present moment and the nonjudgmental aspect of mindfulness. Mindfulness is an innate human capacity to deliberately pay full attention to where we are, to our actual experience, and to learn from it. This can be contrasted with living on automatic pilot and going through our day without really being there. We can drive to work or take a shower and not be there for it. Everyone is familiar with the experience of driving somewhere and suddenly realizing that they were hardly aware of driving, not even knowing in that instant where they are.

Thich Nhat Hanh, a Vietnamese Zen monk, poet, and peacemaker summarized the essence of mindfulness in a radio interview:

Mindfulness is a part of living. When you are mindful, you are fully alive, you are fully present. You can get in touch with the wonders of life that can nourish you and heal you. And you are stronger, you are more solid in order to handle the suffering inside of you and around you. When you are mindful, you can recognize, embrace and handle the pain, the sorrow in you and around you. . . . And if you continue with concentration and insight, you'll be able to transform the suffering inside and help transform the suffering around you. (transcript available at *speakingoffaith.publicradio.org/programs/thichnhathanh/transcript.shtml*)

The practice of mindfulness involves both formal and informal meditation practices and nonmeditation-based exercises. Formal mindfulness, most often referred to as meditation, involves intense introspection whereby one sustains one's attention on an object (breath, body sensations) or on whatever arises in each moment (called choiceless awareness). Informal mindfulness is the application of mindful attention in everyday life. Mindful eating and mindful walking are examples of informal mindfulness practices. In fact any daily activity can be the object of informal mindfulness practice. In my mindfulness classes I engage people early on with informal practice, asking them to mindfully undertake one activity each day between classes and report on the experience. The list of activities they report is endless: mindfully brushing the teeth, mindful driving behind a slow car, mindful ironing, and so forth.

Nonmeditation-based mindfulness exercises are specifically used in dialectical behavior therapy (DBT; Linehan, 1993) and acceptance and commitment therapy (ACT; Hayes, Strosahl, & Wilson, 1999; see below). Therapists and therapist trainers could use some of these exercises to cultivate mindfulness for their therapeutic relationships. ACT involves 41 exercises, nine of which are of the formal or informal mindfulness type. The remainder are not meditation based. For example, ACT begins with an exercise called "your suffering inventory" whereby the client lists and ranks painful and difficult issues in his or her life. Another exercise displays how difficult it is to suppress our thoughts. It asks participants to get a clear picture of a yellow jeep in their minds and then try as hard as they can not to think even one single thought about a yellow jeep. DBT involves extensive questionnaires and exercises to assist clients in better regulating emotions, increase their sense of personal identity, and sharpen their judgment and observation skills. Other practices involve paying attention to environmental elements such as music or aromas (Baer, 2006).

Whether meditation based or not, mindfulness is an ongoing discipline and practice that refines our capacity for paying attention, and it is this that provides the potential for effective therapeutic relationships. One often begins mindfulness training by simplifying and narrowing one's focus of attention to something, for example the breath or a particular activity. Intentionally observing something like the breath, a feature of life that is almost always taken for granted, one begins to train the mind in mindfulness. By simply feeling the sensations of the breath entering and leaving the body one can practice being in the present moment. It sound like a simple exercise, but trying it reveals how difficult it actually is to do. The mind will wander off, thinking about what happened yesterday or planning the afternoon.

Mindfulness is a nonstriving activity. It isn't about getting anywhere or attaining any special state of mind—even relaxation or stress relief. This presents an interesting paradox for practitioners offering mindfulness courses for stress reduction or symptom management. People come to the course with expectations and the desire for results and are told, usually in the first session, to put aside those goals and just let things be, resting in awareness, observing the mind, body, and world unfolding in the present moment. It can also be a challenge for people in our results-oriented society.

MINDFULNESS APPLICATIONS AND PRACTICES

Most mindfulness research has been conducted within the area of mindfulness-based interventions. Although this book is not directly concerned with mindfulness-based interventions and their effectiveness, they provide a useful context for the discussion of mindfulness as a way of cultivating a positive therapeutic relationship and for teaching how to do this.

Mindfulness has been used in wide variety of clinical and therapeutic settings, having been shown to be effective with chronic pain (Kabat-Zinn, 1984, 1990; Kabat-Zinn, Lipworth, Burney, & Sellers, 1987), stress (Shapiro, Schwartz, & Bonner, 1998), depressive relapse (Segal et al., 2002; Teasdale et al., 2000), disordered eating (Kristeller & Hallett, 1999), cancer (Monti et al., 2006; Carlson, Ursuliak, Goodey, Angen, & Speca, 2001), and suicidal behavior (Linehan, Armstrong, Suarez, Allman, & Heard, 1991; Williams, Duggan, Crane, & Fennell, 2006). In their overview of mindfulness-based interventions, Salmon, Santorelli, and Kabat-Zinn (1998) documented 240 programs. Baer (2003, 2006) provides a review of mindfulness-based interventions.

The first of the mindfulness-based interventions was MBSR (Kabat-

Zinn, 1990). The core program of MBSR consists of eight weekly 2- to 3-hour classes and one daylong class. It includes formal guided instruction in mindfulness meditation and mindful body movement or yoga practices, exercises to enhance awareness in everyday life, daily assignments lasting from 45 minutes to an hour that are largely meditations, and methods for improving communication. The program emphasizes being present with sensations within the body, and then expanding this to emotions and thoughts. MBSR aims to help people develop an ongoing meditation practice. Participants are provided with two CDs, each containing four or five guided meditations.

More recently, mindfulness-based cognitive therapy (MBCT) was developed as a treatment approach to reduce relapse and recurrence of depression (Segal et al., 2002). Two controlled clinical trials demonstrated that MBCT can reduce the likelihood of relapse by between 40 and 50% in people who have suffered three or more previous episodes of depression (Kenny & Williams, 2007; Ma & Teasdale, 2004; Teasdale et al., 2000). MBCT is based on MBSR, but integrates several elements of cognitive therapy such as client education and emphasis on the role of negative thoughts, and on how rumination, avoidance, suppression, and the struggle with unhelpful cognitions and emotions can perpetuate distress rather than resolve it (Williams et al., 2006, p. 202). That said, MBCT does differ substantially from cognitive therapy. MBCT emphasizes the acceptance of thoughts as thoughts rather than strategies to change the content of thinking. Instead of learning to replace negative thoughts with positive thoughts, MBCT focuses on noticing the effects of negative thoughts on the body in terms of body sensations. Mark Williams and his team at the University of Oxford are exploring the use of MBCT with suicidal individuals (Williams et al., 2006).

The practices contained in mindfulness-based interventions include a variety of exercises or meditations for building awareness and compassion. MBSR and MBCT emphasize formal guided meditations combined with informal mindful living exercises. ACT and DBT emphasize nonmeditation based activities and exercises but include some meditation.

OPERATIONAL DEFINITIONS AND MEASURES OF MINDFULNESS

Researchers, primarily within psychology, have recently endeavored to specify their definitions of mindfulness. This has occurred at two levels. First, discussions have been tightened and clarified. Secondly, at least eight quantitative measures of mindfulness have been developed and tested. Surprisingly, at least to me, there is little critique of this trend toward instrumentalizing mindfulness. In other social science research areas, positivist and instrumentalist approaches would be critiqued.

With these cautions in mind, I next review the attempts at defining and measuring mindfulness. Dimidjian and Linehan have worked toward precision in refining their definition of mindfulness as involving three qualities and three activities (2003, p. 166). The three qualities include (1) observing, noticing, bringing awareness; (2) describing, labeling, and noting; and (3) participating. The accompanying activities are (1) nonjudgmentally, with acceptance, allowing; (2) in the present moment, with beginner's mind; and (3) effectively. This is a complex definition that captures the key components of mindfulness. In a similar attempt to operationalize mindfulness, Bishop et. al. (2004, p. 230) see mindfulness as comprising two main components. The first component is metacognitive skills, which involve sustained self-regulated attention, attention switching, and the inhibition of elaborative processing. The second component is one's orientation to the present moment experience. This includes the maintenance of an attitude of curiosity, acceptance of one's experience, and an openness to observe what comes up in the field of awareness.

Shapiro, Carlson, Astin, and Freedman (2006, p. 374) build on Kabat-Zinn's definition of mindfulness as paying attention in a particular way: "on purpose, in the present moment, and non-judgmentally" (Kabat-Zinn, 1994, p. 4). They posit three components (axioms) of mindfulness: (1) intention, (2) attention, and (3) attitude (IAA) as follows:

1. "On purpose" or intention.
2. "Paying attention" or attention.
3. "In a particular way" or attitude (mindfulness qualities).

Building on these components, Shapiro et al. (2006, p. 377) propose a model of the mechanisms of mindfulness, whereby intentionally (I) attending (A) with openness and nonjudgmentalness (A) leads to a significant shift in perspective, which they have termed *reperceiving*. This shift enables people to stand back and simply witness the drama of their lives rather than being immersed in it.

Unlike cognitive therapy's emphasis on "cognitive errors" and "distorted interpretations," mindfulness teaches the practice of observing thoughts without getting entangled in them, approaching them as though they were leaves floating down a stream. It is not about replacing negative thoughts with positive ones, but rather accepting one's ongoing flow of thoughts, sensations, and emotions.

In order to further untangle the impact of the components of mindfulness, several groups have developed scales or measures of mindfulness. At present eight mindfulness measures have been developed. Seven are based on self-reporting of particular trait-like constructs, and one measures mindfulness as a state-like construct. The trait-based measures include the Mindful Attention Awareness Scale (MAAS; Brown & Ryan, 2003), the Freiburg Mindfulness Inventory (FMI; Buchheld, Grossman, & Walach, 2001), the Kentucky Inventory of Mindfulness Skills (KIMS; Baer, Smith, & Allen, 2004), the Cognitive and Affective Mindfulness Scale (CAMS; Feldman, Hayes, Kumar, & Greeson, 2004), the Mindfulness Questionnaire (MQ; Chadwick, Hember, Mead, Lilley, & Dagnan, 2005), the Revised Cognitive and Affective Mindfulness Scale (CAMS-R; Feldman et al., 2004), and the Philadelphia Mindfulness Scale (PHLMS; Cardaciotto, 2005).

The scales tend to measure different aspects of mindfulness and take different approaches. Brown and Ryan's (2003) thoroughly tested MAAS emphasizes measuring attention and awareness but neglects other important aspects of mindfulness such as compassion, nonjudgmental attitude, openness to new experiences, insightful understanding, and nonstriving. The KIMS scale, in contrast, measures qualities and skills taught in DBT. Using a consensus approach, Bishop, Lau, Shapiro, Carlson, Anderson, and Carmody (2004) and 10 colleagues, primarily in Toronto and Calgary, developed the Toronto Mindfulness Scale (TMS; Bishop et al., 2004). This scale takes a different approach and measures mindfulness as a state-like phenomenon (as opposed to a trait-like quality) that is evoked and maintained by regulating attention. Studies have shown that the TMS is a reliable and valid measure useful in investigations of the mediating role of mindful awareness in mindfulness-based interventions (Lau et al., 2006).

RESEARCH ON THE THERAPEUTIC RELATIONSHIP

A key research finding in the past 20 years is that different therapies produce similar positive therapeutic outcomes (Luborsky, Singer, & Luborsky, 1975; Smith & Glass, 1977; Stiles, Shapiro, & Elliott, 1986). As Lambert and Simon indicate in Chapter 2 of this volume, another key finding is that very little of the variance in therapeutic outcomes is due to the treatment model that is used (Lambert, 1992; Lambert & Barley, 2001). This has led researchers to look for elements common to different therapeutic approaches and an analysis of the relationship that forms between therapist and client. Bohart, Elliott, Greenberg, and Watson (2002, p. 96) found that overall, empathy accounts for as much and probably more outcome variance than do specific interventions. Fulton (2005, p. 57) reports that on average 30% of treatment outcome may be attributable to "common factors" that are present in most successful treatment relationships.

The two studies most often cited when discussing the impact of the therapeutic relationship on outcome are both meta-analytic studies (Horvath & Symonds, 1991; Martin, Garske, & Davis, 2000). Horvath and Symonds (1991) found that the therapeutic relationship accounted for moderate amounts of outcome variance, with an average effect size of 0.26. They consider this to be a conservative estimate since any correlations in the 24 studies that were computed but not reported, or were reported but not significant, were treated as zero correlations. Martin et al. (2000) conducted a meta-analysis of 79 studies and found an average effect size of 0.22.

Early explorations of the therapeutic relationship focused solely on the therapist (client-centered) or the client (psychodynamic) as arbiters of the relationship. In the 1970s explorations of the therapeutic relationship focused on the collaborative and interactive elements in the relationship (Bordin, 1979; Luborsky, 1976). Current research is building on the work of Luborsky and Bordin, and there appears to be some agreement that the collaborative work of therapist and client against the client's pain and suffering is central (Bordin, 1979). Researchers are examining different components of the therapeutic relationship, such as the affective relationship between the participants (e.g., warmth, support), specific activities of client and therapist (e.g., self-observation, exploration), negative contributions (e.g., hostility), the sense of partnership or collaboration, and so forth (Bachelor & Horvath, 1999).

While research necessarily isolates variables such as client characteristics and therapist characteristics and treats them as though they were static, independent entities, they are actually best thought of as continuously interacting aspects of an immensely complex interpersonal reality. Miller and Rollnick (2002) suggest, for example, that the trait of denial in alcoholics so often identified by therapists is actually a function of the interpersonal context. Alcoholics are often lectured to by concerned family and friends, and even by therapists of the old school, who hold that their denial must be vigorously confronted. Instead, however, it seems that such treatment actually *elicits* denial, since, like everyone else, alcoholics don't particularly enjoy being lectured to or told what to do. And in fact, they respond better to empathy than to harsh confrontation, as do other human beings.

Summarizing thousands of studies across 60 years, Lambert and Ogles (2004) concluded that variables measuring the effect of the therapeutic relationship consistently correlate more highly with client outcome than specialized therapy techniques. They specify that more successful therapists are more understanding, accepting, empathic, warm, and supportive. Further, they found that therapists who develop positive therapeutic relationships engage less often in negative behaviors such as blaming, ignoring, neglecting, rejecting, or pushing a technique-based agenda when clients are resistant (Lambert & Ogles, 2004).

This is where mindfulness enters the picture. In my own work I have seen mindfulness contribute to the development of the different components of the therapeutic relationship, such as empathy, deep listening, and compassion. Although the research on mindfulness and the therapeutic relationship is in its very early stages, preliminary findings support my anecdotal evidence.

RESEARCH ON MINDFULNESS AND THE CLIENT–THERAPIST RELATIONSHIP

Recently there have been numerous studies on the efficacy of mindfulness interventions for addressing various client difficulties. There is little research examining the impact of mindfulness as training for the therapist and even less on how mindfulness might have an impact on the therapeutic relationship or client outcome via the therapeutic relationship. The focus of mindfulness research has been on the development and testing of "brand-name" mindfulness-based interventions such as MBSR, MBCT, and ACT. The thrust has been to provide evidence that specific mindfulness-based therapeutic techniques are correlated positively with outcome. Further, while MBSR is advertised as a generic approach, recent incarnations of mindfulness-based intervention are oriented more toward manualized approaches to the treatment of specific disorders. This is the case with MBCT, which was explicitly developed for the treatment of depression relapse. As Lambert and Simon suggest in Chapter 2, the emphasis within the mindfulness research may be misplaced. They argue that if research on mindfulness as an intervention strategy follows the trajectory of research on other psychotherapy techniques, then ultimately it will reveal that the intervention plays only a small role in positive outcome—the larger share of outcome being attributable to common factors such as the therapeutic relationship.

In other psychotherapy treatments, Norcross (2002, p. 5) found, specific techniques account for only 5–15% of the outcome variance. The remainder is attributed to circumstances outside the control of therapy or relationship factors. If the same holds true for mindfulness-based interventions, and there is little reason to doubt this, then we may be missing an important piece of the outcome puzzle. In addition, if mindfulness is viewed as a way of being in the world rather than an instrumental set of methods, then perhaps relationship is even more important. After all, relationships are mostly about the way we are with another person or persons. Mindfulness guides us in how to be deeply present with ourselves and others. In my mind, mindfulness is about cultivating, sustaining, and integrating a way of paying attention to the ebb and flow of emotions, thoughts, and perceptions within all human beings. This kind of awareness can enable us as therapists, community workers, or group counselors to be present in a therapeutic relationship in a different way—a way that is more about being with clients than about being a detached expert.

Discussions about mindfulness-based interventions generally examine what is being taught to clients, but what about the therapists themselves? Most, if not all, discussions about mindfulness-based interventions strongly suggest that the people who teach the programs should practice mindfulness themselves, in a "practice what you preach" model. However, thus far there is little evidence on this aspect of the practice.

In one of the few studies of mindfulness and the therapeutic relationship, Wexler (2006) used a correlational design to examine the relationship between therapist mindfulness and the quality of the therapeutic alliance. Therapist mindfulness was measured using the MAAS (Brown & Ryan, 2003), and the therapeutic alliance was measured using dyadic ratings from the Working Alliance Inventory (WAI; Horvath & Greenberg, 1989). Data from a sample of 19 therapist–client dyads revealed significant positive correlations between both client and therapist perception of the alliance and therapist mindfulness, both in and out of therapy.

Grepmair et al. (2007a, 2007b) performed what is perhaps the first controlled large-scale study of the effects of mindfulness in psychotherapists in training on treatment results. They examined the therapeutic treatment course and results of 124 inpatients using a randomized, double-blind controlled study. They compared the outcomes for 18 different therapists, nine of whom undertook a 9-week mediation course and nine who did not meditate at all. They found that compared to the group with nonmeditating therapists ($n = 61$), the inpatients of the mediators ($n = 63$) was significantly higher using a variety of scales. Furthermore they found that the inpatients of the mediators showed greater symptom reduction, better assessments of their progress in overcoming their difficulties, greater rate of change, and higher subjectively perceived results.

A few other studies have directly examined the impact of mindfulness practices on the cultivation of empathy within practitioners (Aiken, 2006; Shapiro et al., 1998; Wang, 2006). Shapiro et al. (1998) assessed the efficacy of a short-term mindfulness-based intervention in enhancing the doctor–patient relationship through the cultivation of empathy. Using the 42-item Empathy Construct Rating Scale (ECRS) to provide a measure of empathy, the 200 medical students who received mindfulness training showed significant increased levels of empathy, with an alpha coefficient of .89.

In another study, Wang (2006) measured the impact of mindfulness meditation on specific relationship variables such as psychotherapists' levels of awareness or attention and empathy. Two groups of psychotherapists (meditators versus nonmeditators) were compared using measures of awareness or attention, and empathy. Eight meditating psychotherapists also participated in semistructured interviews. The study found no significant differences between meditating psychotherapists and nonmeditating psychotherapists on the attention or awareness levels. However, meditating psychotherapists scored significantly higher levels of empathy than nonmeditating psychotherapists. Qualitative data also supported enhanced levels of attention and awareness, empathy, nonjudgmental acceptance, love, and compassion.

Qualitative interviews (Aiken, 2006) with six psychotherapy practitioners with extensive mindfulness practice (over 10 years) found that mindfulness contributes to a therapist's ability to achieve a felt sense of the client's inner experience; communicate his or her awareness of that felt sense; be more present to the pain and suffering of the client; and help clients become better able to be present to and give language to their bodily feelings and sensations. Aiken (2006) examined how mindfulness practice may have noticeable effects on a therapist's ability to cultivate an empathic orientation.

While containing obvious limitations, this research is promising, illustrating the potential effects of practitioner mindfulness on the therapeutic relationship. It is important to note that a study by Stratton (2005) did not support a correlation between therapist mindfulness and general client outcomes. The study measured mindfulness of the therapist using the MAAS and the Mindfulness/Mindlessness Scale (MMS), and this was correlated with client outcome scores as measured by the Outcome Questionnaire 45 (OQ-45). While this study did not directly measure the impact of mindfulness on the therapeutic relationship or its variables, it does highlight the need for further study.

Future research is needed to explore the impacts and effects of mindfulness on therapists and the therapeutic relationship, and then ultimately on client outcome.

CONCLUSION

Teasdale, Segal, and Williams (2003, p. 158) maintain that the way in which mindfulness training is delivered may be as important as the content of what is delivered. Others (Bien, 2006; Epstein, 1995; Linehan, 1993) have recognized that mindfulness, while generally conceptualized as an intervention, should also be examined as a therapeutic strategy—as attitudes and behaviors that a therapist demonstrates as opposed to skills that are taught to clients. As we will see in Chapter 2, what the therapist communicates has a lot to do with the therapeutic relationship.

Bishop et al. (2004) report that in a mindful state, practitioners are better able to observe thoughts, feelings, and sensations dispassionately and without attachment. This dispassionate state of self-observation, according to Bishop et al., may introduce a delay between one's perception and response. Mindfulness may therefore enable practitioners to respond to situations more reflectively.

Thomas Bien (2006, p. 217), in his book *Mindful Therapy*, observes that to him "mindful therapy is therapy in which the therapist produces true presence and deep listening. It is not technique driven." This insight reflects the importance Bien attaches to the role of mindfulness in cultivating presence and listening within the client–therapist relationship. But he also sees the role of mindfulness in another light. His book is as much about the therapeutic relationship as it is about how therapists can use mindfulness to take better care of themselves. This aspect of mindfulness as self-care has the potential to positively affect the therapist and in turn the therapeutic relationship.

REFERENCES

Aiken, G. A. (2006). *The potential effect of mindfulness meditation on the cultivation of empathy in psychotherapy.* PhD thesis, Saybrook Graduate School and Research Center, San Francisco, CA.

Bachelor, A., & Horvath, A. (1999). The therapeutic relationship. In M. A. Hubble, B. L.

Duncan, & S. D. Miller (Eds.), *The heart and soul of change: What works in therapy* (pp. 133–178). Washington, DC: American Psychological Association.

Baer, R. A. (2003). Mindfulness training as a clinical intervention: A conceptual and empirical review. *Clinical Psychology: Science and Practice, 10*(2), 125–142.

Baer, R. A. (Ed.). (2006). *Mindfulness-based treatment approaches: Clinician's guide to evidence base and applications.* Burlington, MA: Academic Press.

Baer, R. A., Smith, G. T., & Allen, K. B. (2004). Assessment of mindfulness by self-report: The Kentucky Inventory of Mindfulness Skills. *Assessment, 11,* 191–206.

Bien, T. (2006). *Mindful therapy: A guide for therapists and helping professionals.* Boston: Wisdom.

Bishop, S., Lau, M., Shapiro, S., Carlson, L., Anderson, N., & Carmody, J. (2004). Mindfulness: A proposed operational definition. *Clinical Psychology: Science and Practice, 11,* 230–241.

Bohart, A. C., Elliott, R., Greenberg, L. S., & Watson, J. C. (2002). Empathy. In J. C. Norcorss (Ed.), *Psychotherapy relationships that work: Therapist contributions and responsiveness to clients* (pp. 89–108). New York: Oxford University Press.

Bordin, E. S. (1979). The generalizability of the psychoanalytic concept of the working alliance. *Psychotherapy: Theory, Research, and Practice, 16,* 252–260.

Brandon, D. (1976). *Zen in the art of helping,* London: Penguin Books.

Brown, K. W., & Ryan, R. M. (2003). The benefits of being present: Mindfulness and its role in psychological well-being. *Journal of Personality and Social Psychology, 84,* 822–848.

Buchheld, N., Grossman, P., & Walach, H. (2001). Measuring mindfulness in insight meditation (Vipassana) and meditation-based psychotherapy: The development of the Freiburg Mindfulness Inventory (FMI). *Journal for Meditation and Meditation Research, 1,* 11–34.

Cardaciotto, L. (2005). *Assessing mindfulness: The development of a bi-dimensional measure of awareness and acceptance.* Unpublished manuscript, Drexel University, Philadelphia.

Carlson, L. E., Ursuliak, Z., Goodey, E., Angen, M., & Speca, M. (2001). The effects of a mindfulness meditation-based stress reduction program on mood and symptoms of stress in cancer outpatients: 6-month follow-up. *Support Care Cancer, 9,* 112–123.

Chadwick, P., Hember, M., Mead, S., Lilley, B., & Dagnan, D. (2005). *Responding mindfully to unpleasant thoughts and images: Reliability and validity of the Mindfulness Questionnaire.* Manuscript under review.

Dimidjian, S., & Linehan, M. M. (2003). Defining an agenda for future research on the clinical applications of mindfulness practice. *Clinical Psychology: Science and Practice, 10*(2), 166–171.

Epstein, M. (1995). *Thoughts without a thinker.* New York: Basic Books.

Feldman, G. C., Hayes. A. M., Kumar, S. M., & Greeson, J. M. (2004). *Development, factor structure, and initial validation of the Cognitive and Affective Mindfulness Scale.* Manuscript submitted for publication.

Fulton, P. R. (2005). Mindfulness as clinical training. In C. K. Germer, R. D. Siegel, & P. R. Fulton (Eds.), *Mindfulness and psychotherapy* (pp. 55–72). New York: Guilford Press.

Grepmair, L., Mitterlehner, F., Loew, T., Bachler, E., Rother, W., & Nickel, M. (2007a). Promoting mindfulness in psychotherapists in training influences the treatment results of their patients: A randomized, double-blind, controlled study. *Psychotherapy and Psychosomatics, 76,* 332–338.

Grepmair, L., Loew, T., Bachler, E., Rother, W., & Nickel, M. (2007b). Promotion of mindfulness in psychotherapists in training: Preliminary study. *European Psychiatry, 22*(8), 485–489.

Hayes, S. C., Strosahl, K. D., & Wilson, K. G. (1999). *Acceptance and commitment therapy.* New York: Guilford Press.

Horvath, A. O., & Greenberg, L. S. (1989). Development and validation of the Working Alliance Inventory. *Journal of Counseling Psychology, 36*(2), 223–233.

Horvath, A. O., & Symonds, B. D. (1991). Relation between working alliance and outcome in psychotherapy: A meta-analysis. *Journal of Counseling Psychology, 38*, 139–149.

Kabat-Zinn, J. (1984). An outpatient program in behavioral medicine for chronic pain patients based in the practice of mindfulness meditation: Theoretical considerations and preliminary results. *General Hospital Psychiatry, 4*, 33–47.

Kabat-Zinn, J. (1990). *Full catastrophe living: Using the wisdom of your body and mind to face stress, pain, and illness.* New York: Dell.

Kabat-Zinn, J. (1994). *Wherever you go there you are: Mindfulness meditation in everyday life.* New York: Hyperion.

Kabat-Zinn, J., Lipworth, L., Burney, R., & Sellers, W. (1987). Four-year follow-up of a meditation based program for the self-regulation of chronic pain: Treatment outcomes and compliance. *Clinical Journal of Pain, 2*, 159–173.

Kenny, M. A., & Williams, J. M. G. (2007). Treatment-resistant depressed patients show a good response to mindfulness-based cognitive therapy. *Behaviour Research and Therapy, 45*, 617–625.

Kristeller, J. L., & Hallett, B. (1999). Effects of a meditation-based intervention in the treatment of binge eating. *Journal of Health Psychology, 4*, 357–363.

Lambert, M. J. (1992). Implications of outcome research for psychotherapy integration. In J. C. Norcross & M. R. Goldstein (Eds.), *The handbook of psychology integration* (pp. 94–129). New York: Basic Books.

Lambert, M. J., & Barley, D. E. (2001). Research summary on the therapeutic relationship and psychotherapy outcome. *Psychotherapy, 38*(4), 357–361.

Lambert, M. J., & Ogles, B. M. (2004). The efficacy and effectiveness of psychotherapy. In M. J. Lambert (Ed.), *Bergin and Garfield's handbook of psychotherapy and behavior change* (5th ed., pp. 139–193). New York: Wiley.

Lau, M. A., Bishop, S. R., Segal, S. V., Buis, T., Anderson, N. D., Carlson, L., et al. (2006). The Toronto Mindfulness Scale: Development and validation. *Journal of Clinical Psychology, 62*(12), 1445–1467.

Linehan, M. M. (1993). *Cognitive-behavioral treatment of borderline personality disorder.* New York: Guilford Press.

Linehan, M. M., Armstrong, H. E., Suarez, A., Allmon, D., & Heard, H. L. (1991). Cognitive-behavioral treatment of chronically parasuicidal borderline patients. *Archives of General Psychiatry, 48*, 1060–1064.

Luborsky, L. (1976). Helping alliances in psychotherapy. In J. L. Cleghorn (Ed.), *Successful psychotherapy* (pp. 92–116). New York: Brunner/Mazel.

Luborsky, L., Singer, B., & Luborsky, L. (1975). Comparative studies of psychotherapies: Is it true that "Everyone has won and all must have prizes"? *Archives of General Psychiatry, 32*, 995–1008.

Ma, S. H., & Teasdale, J. D. (2004). Mindfulness-based cognitive therapy for depression: Replication and exploration of differential relapse prevention effects. *Journal of Consulting and Clinical Psychology, 72*, 31–40.

Martin, D. J., Garske, J. P., & Davis, M. K. (2000). Relation of therapeutic alliance with outcome and other variables: A meta-analytic review. *Journal of Consulting and Clinical Psychology, 68*, 438–450.

Miller, W. R., & Rollnick, S. (2002). *Motivational interviewing: Preparing people for change* (2nd ed.). New York: Guilford Press.

Monti, D. A., Peterson, C., Shakin Kunkel, E. J., Hauck, W. W., Pequignot, E., Rhodes, L., et al. (2006). A randomized, controlled trial of mindfulness-based art therapy (MBAT) for women with cancer. *Psycho-Oncology, 15*(5), 363–373.

Norcross, J. C. (2002). *Psychotherapy relationships that work: Therapist contributions and responsiveness to clients.* New York: Oxford University Press.

Rosenberg, L. (1998). *Breath by breath: The liberating practice of insight meditation.* Boston: Shambhala Press.

Salmon, P. G., Santorelli, S. F., & Kabat-Zinn, J. (1998). Intervention elements in promoting adherence to mindfulness-based stress reduction programs in the clinical behavioral medicine setting. In S. A. Shumaker, E. B. Schron, J. K. Ockene, & W. L. Bee (Eds.), *Handbook of health behavior change* (2nd ed., pp. 239–268). New York: Springer.

Saunders, S. M., Howard, K. I., & Orlinsky, D. E. (1989). The therapeutic bond scales: Psychometric characteristics and relationship to treatment effectiveness. *Psychological Assessment, 1,* 323–330.

Segal, Z. V., Williams, J. M. G., & Teasdale, J. D. (2002). *Mindfulness-based cognitive therapy for depression: A new approach to preventing relapse.* New York: Guilford Press.

Shapiro, S. L., Carlson, L. E., Astin, J. A., & Freedman, B. (2006). Mechanisms of mindfulness. *Journal of Clinical Psychology, 62*(3), 373–386.

Shapiro, S. L., Schwartz, G. E., & Bonner, G. (1998). Effects of mindfulness-based stress reduction on medical or premedical students. *Journal of Behavioral Medicine, 21,* 581–599.

Smith, M. L., & Glass, G. U. (1977). Meta-analysis of psychotherapy outcome studies. *American Psychologist, 32,* 752–760.

Stiles, W. B., Shapiro, D., & Elliot, R. (1986). Are all psychotherapies equivalent? *American Psychologist, 41,* 165–180.

Stratton, P. (2005). *Therapist mindfulness as a predictor of client outcomes.* Unpublished manuscript, Capella University, Minneapolis, MN.

Teasdale, J. D., Segal, Z. V., & Williams, J. M. G. (2003). Mindfulness training and problem formulation. *Clinical Psychology: Science and Practice, 10*(2), 157–160.

Teasdale, J. D., Segal, Z. V., Williams, J. M. G., Ridgeway, V. A., Soulsby, J., & Lau, M. A. (2000). Prevention of relapse/recurrence in major depression by mindfulness-based cognitive therapy. *Journal of Consulting and Clinical Psychology, 68,* 615–623.

Varela, F. J., Thompson, E., & Rosch, E. (1991). *The embodied mind: Cognitive science and human experience.* Cambridge, MA: MIT Press.

Wang, S. J. (2006). *Mindfulness meditation: Its personal and professional impact on psychotherapists.* Unpublished manuscript, Capella University, Minneapolis, MN.

Wexler, J. (2006). *The relationship between therapist mindfulness and the therapeutic alliance.* Unpublished manuscript, Massachusetts School of Professional Psychology, Boston, MA.

Wheat, P. (2005, January). Mindfulness meditation: Promoting cultural competency. *Spectrum,* pp. 18–19.

Williams, J. M., Duggan, D. S., Crane, C., & Fennell, M. J. V. (2006). Mindfulness-based cognitive therapy for prevention of recurrence of suicidal behavior. *Journal of Clinical Psychology, 62*(2), 201–210.

2 The Therapeutic Relationship

*Central and Essential
in Psychotherapy Outcome*

MICHAEL J. LAMBERT
WITOLD SIMON

Among the most consistent findings of psychotherapy outcome research is that the therapeutic relationship is vital in contributing to client progress. Even recent technological developments in neuroscience support the importance of developing and maintaining a therapeutic relationship through activation of areas of the brain related to the attachment system (Fonagy, 2006). This chapter briefly summarizes conceptions and theoretical underpinnings of the therapy relationship, highlights empirical research that strongly supports the centrality of the therapeutic relationship as a primary factor contributing to psychotherapy outcome, makes suggestions for studying the therapeutic relationship in relation to mindfulness, and encourages systematically tracking the quality of the relationship in mindfulness interventions.

Research on psychotherapy outcome has examined the relationship between a host of variables and client progress. Such variables include *client factors* such as the severity, chronicity, and complexity of the condition, the presence of underlying personality problems, and diagnosis. In addition, considerable research has investigated *extratherapeutic factors* such as negative life events and social supports. Positive outcomes have also been linked with *factors common* to all treatments (variables found in most therapies regardless of the treatment techniques), such as client and therapist expectancy of a positive outcome (e.g., the client's belief in the treatment techniques and rationale), provision of expert guided care, a supportive human encounter, motivation (e.g., readiness to accept responsibility for problem solution), and attention from the therapist, as well as the client–therapist relationship. As important as these factors are, treatment specific variables and a host of therapy specific actions, including particular techniques like challenging cognitive distortions, are believed by many to be the central curative factor, and they play the central role in the clinical trial research that provides the foundation for evidence-based practices. Despite advocacy of empirically supported psychotherapy by the American Psychological Association and other professional groups (American Psychological Association, 2006), it is likely that common factors play a much larger role in restoring client functioning than specific theory-based techniques (Lambert & Ogles, 2004; Wampold, 2001). Among the common factors that have an especially well-documented place in enhancing client outcome is the quality of the client–therapist relationship, one of the central features of the "common factors" explanation of change. Below we present, a brief history of the theory and measurement of the client–therapist relationship and methods of studying it in order to place more recent findings about its importance in context.

CONCEPTUAL AND METHODOLOGICAL ISSUES

The profound importance of relationships in the healing of mental patients on the therapeutic journey was noted by Freud (1913/1958) as psychotherapy was just beginning to emerge as a healing technique. Different aspects of the relationship were noted in psychoanalysis (e.g., the real relationship, transference, and therapeutic alliance; Greenson, 1965; Meissner, 2006). The concept of therapeutic alliance—considered as a phenomenon shared by the patient and the analyst—has made a distinctive contribution to the psychoanalytic theory of patient–analyst interactions aimed at fostering the collaborative relationship process (Ponsi, 2000).

A major conceptual shift in emphasis of the therapeutic relationship as a healing force came forth by the early 1960s. This change is notable for its focus on the "real" (as opposed to transference elements of the client–therapist encounter. Rogers (1957) and his colleagues stressed the healing properties of therapist-provided facilitative conditions, attitudes characterized by empathic understanding (the degree to which the therapist is successful in communicating awareness and understanding of the client's current experience in language that is attuned to that client); nonpossessive warmth and positive regard (the extent to which the therapist communicates nonevaluative caring and respect for the client as a person); and congruence (the extent to which the therapist is nondefensive, real, and "non-phony" in interactions with the client). They stressed the importance of valuing the client and entering the therapy relationship without the "comfort of a protective cloak of professional authority" (Thorne, 1992, p. 45). The client–therapist interaction was considered essential for relief and growth, with the client's perception of the therapist the essential component.

In published research the client-centered operational conception of the therapeutic relationship was replaced by renewed efforts to discuss the relationship in terms of the working or therapeutic alliance with research scales largely informed by psychodynamic formulations, but in a format intended to be pantheoretical enough to be applicable to all psychotherapy. Measures that developed from these research groups, such as Horvath and Greenberg's (1994) Working Alliance Inventory (WAI), and Luborsky's (1994) Helping Alliance Questionnaire, attempted to assess the degree to which client and therapist concur on the purposes of their work together, but also on the way such goals are to be achieved. These measures also include items that attempt to capture the attachment between therapist and client—the mutual trust, confidence, and acceptance (the affective bond). The therapist's contribution to the alliance, such as the ability to come to a mutual agreement with the client on the goals of treatment, is also measured (Hatcher & Barends, 1996).

In a positive alliance both the therapist and the client view the therapy as important and relevant. In an alliance that is less than ideal the working partners find one or more of the alliance factors are diminished (e.g., the client may feel there is a positive bond and agree with the therapist about desirable end states but feel that the way time is spent in session is not optimally helpful or relevant). A poor alliance may lead to deterioration in terms of symptoms, poorer interpersonal functioning, and, eventually, premature therapy termination (dropout) (Gajowy, Marchewka, Sala, & Simon, 2004).

Of course many researchers, rather than assuming they already knew what was important in determining outcome, endeavored to provide open-ended questions following each session or, more broadly, to ask for client retrospective reflection long after treatment ended. For example, Murphy, Cramer, and Lillie (1984) had outpatients list curative factors that they believed to be associated with successful cognitive-behavioral therapy (CBT). The factors endorsed by a significant portion of patients were advice (79%), "talking to someone interested in my problems" (75%), encouragement and reassurance (67%), "talking to someone who understands" (58%), and instillation of hope (58%). The two factors that correlated most highly with outcome, as assessed by both therapist and client, were "talking to someone who understands" and "receiving advice." The point to be made here is that neither the client-centered literature nor that on the therapeutic alliance is sufficient to characterize the broader concept of the therapeutic relationship. We attempt to discuss the therapeutic relationship more broadly here and begin with an examination of the individual therapist and relationship issues.

SUMMARY OF RESEARCH
AND ITS IMPLICATIONS FOR MINDFULNESS

Therapist Attributes and Facilitative Conditions

In controlled studies the independent variable of interest is the kind of psychotherapy or intervention technique. In such circumstances major efforts are expended to eliminate the therapist as a causal contributor to client improvement. Despite such attempts variability in outcome is more strongly associated with therapists rather than type of treatment. This finding is consistent across numerous studies (e.g., Luborsky, McClellan, Woody, O'Brien, & Auerbach, 1985; Okiishi et al., 2006). Lazarus (1971), for example, noted in an uncontrolled follow-up of 112 clients he had treated with multimodal therapy that they chose adjectives such as "sensitive," "gentle," and "honest" to describe him and made almost no reference to the techniques he used, though these were viewed by Lazarus as essential to their improvement. Similarly, Strupp, Fox, and Lessler (1969) reported that patients who felt that their therapy was successful described their therapist as "warm, attentive, interested, understanding, and respectful" (p. 116). Ricks (1974) published an in-depth naturalistic case study of two therapists working with a group of equally disturbed adolescent boys to identify what better therapists do. Differences in outcome were attributed to the differences in the two therapists' styles of interaction with the clients. The therapist whose patients had the better outcome spent more time with the difficult cases, made use of resources outside the immediate therapy circumstances, was firm and direct with parents, encouraged autonomy, implemented problem-solving skills, and had strong therapeutic relationships.

Miller, Taylor, and West (1980) collected data on the contribution of therapist empathy to patient outcome. At the 6- to 8-month follow-up interviews, client ratings of therapist empathy correlated significantly (r = .82) with client outcome, thus accounting for 67% of the variance on the criteria. These results argue for the importance of therapist empathy, even within behavioral and other technique-centered interventions. In another illustrative study, Lafferty, Beutler, and Crago (1991) examined effectiveness of trainee psychotherapists. Outcome was determined by client self-ratings on the SCL-90-R. The less effective therapists were shown to have low levels of empathic understanding: "Clients of less effective therapists felt less understood by their therapists than did clients of more effective therapists" (p. 79).

Lorr (1965) requested that 523 psychotherapy patients describe their therapists with 65 different statements. A factor analysis identified the following five therapist descriptions as factors: understanding, accepting, authoritarian (directive), independence–encouraging, and critical–hostile. Clients' ratings on the understanding and accepting factors correlated most highly with client and therapist-rated improvement. In Elliott, Clark, and Kemeny's (1991) study the highest ratings by clients and therapists were given to feeling understood, self-awareness, and feeling close to or being supported by the therapist.

Similar findings have been reported by Howgego, Yellowlees, Owen, Meldrum, and Dark (2003), who examined the evidence supporting the assumed link between a positive therapeutic alliance and a positive outcome for patients with a mental illness who were managed in community mental health services by case managers. She concluded that the alliance predicted outcome for patients engaged in case management services and suggested that focus on the relationship helped therapists work with persons with serious mentally illness to optimize their strengths in the community.

We hope these examples help the reader appreciate that the therapeutic relationship can be defined in a myriad of ways and that individual therapists make an important contribution to its quality. Before turning to the implications for mindfulness interventions we briefly summarize more traditional methodologies that characterize research directly related to the client-centered and therapeutic alliance literature.

Many older reviews have tried to summarize the relationship between the facilitative conditions proposed by the person-centered school and client outcomes (e.g. Lambert, DeJulio, & Stein, 1978; Parloff, Waskow, & Wolfe; 1978; Truax, 1971). These reviews have suggested a modest relationship between such factors as accurate empathy, warmth, and genuineness and measures of outcome, with the largest correlations coming from client ratings of the relationship (rather than the perceptions of objective raters or therapists) and client self-reports of outcome. From the number of studies that have been reviewed, we can be confident that the relationship between client-centered variables and outcome at the end of therapy is firmly established. Since the experimental manipulation of relationship conditions by the therapist would be highly unethical, no cause–effect conclusions from experimental studies can be drawn from this literature.

Therapeutic Alliance and Outcome

Investigators who espouse psychodynamic theories have produced most of the research on the therapeutic alliance (Gaston, 1990; Horvath & Greenberg, 1994; Horvath & Luborsky, 1993; Luborsky, 1994). However, the therapeutic alliance has also received considerable emphasis in investigations of behavioral and cognitive-behavioral therapy (DeRubeis & Feeley, 1991; Castonguay, Goldfried, Wiser, Raue, & Hayes, 1996), gestalt therapy (Horvath & Greenberg, 1989), and person-centered therapy (Grawe, Caspar, & Ambuhl, 1990). The therapeutic alliance has been measured by client ratings, therapist ratings, and judges' ratings. Specialized self-reports have been created for couple therapy (Mamodhoussen, 2005), mental health centers (McGuire-Snieckus, 2007), physical medicine (Van der Feltz-Cornelis, 2004), and group therapy (Johnson, Burlingame, Olsen, Davies, & Gleave, 2006). These later scales may have special relevance to mindfulness since mindfulness interventions are often delivered in a group therapy format.

There are now widely accepted methods for measuring therapeutic alliance and outcome (Gaston, 1990), but the proliferation of measures makes integration of findings difficult. Many of the measures overlap, but important differences can also be detected (Horvath & Bedi, 2002). While measures of the facilitative conditions typically focus only on the therapist's behaviors, conceptualizations and measures of the therapeutic alliance also emphasize client variables, mainly the client's ability to participate in therapy. Because of their increased scope alliance measures would be expected to correlate more highly with client outcome than measures of facilitative conditions.

Reviews of the research (Gaston, 1990; Horvath & Greenberg, 1994; Horvath & Luborsky, 1993; Martin, Garske, & Davis, 2000) have reported a positive relationship between the therapeutic alliance and outcome across studies, even though there are instances where the alliance fails to predict outcome, or where associations are not significant. Safran and Wallner (1991) studied a sample of 22 outpatients who received time-limited cognitive therapy. The therapeutic alliance was measured using the WAI and the California Psychotherapy Alliance Scale (CALPAS). Results indicated that both measures were predictive of outcome when administered after the third session. These findings underscore the importance of the alliance in CBT and are consistent with research indicating that therapy outcome can be predicted by ratings of the therapeutic alliance in the early stages of treatment (Horvath & Luborsky, 1993).

Castonguay and colleagues (1996) compared the impact of the treatment variable unique to cognitive therapy (the therapist's focus on distorted cognition and depressive symptoms) and two variables common with other forms of treatment (the therapeutic alliance and client emotional involvement) on treatment outcome. Participants were 30 clients suffering from major depressive disorder who received either cognitive therapy alone or cognitive therapy with medication over a 12-week period. Results revealed that the therapeutic alliance and the clients' emotional experience were both found to be positively related to client improvement. In contrast, the variable deemed to be distinctive to cognitive therapy, connecting distorted thoughts to unwanted emotion, was positively correlated to depressive symptoms following therapy (i.e., higher depression). The authors proposed that this finding could have been due to the therapists' efforts to mend the therapeutic alliance through trying to convince the client to accept the legitimacy of the cognitive therapy approach or by viewing alliance difficulties as evidence of the client's distorted cognitions that required disputation. Such actions would not be expected to increase a client's experience of being understood and accepted.

Looking across thousands of studies across 60 years, the implications of relationship research for successful psychotherapy seem clear. Psychotherapy is successful in general, and the average treated client is better off than 80% of untreated controls. Comparative studies of psychotherapy techniques report the relative equivalence of therapies in promoting client change. Measures of therapeutic relationship variables consistently correlate more highly with client outcome than specialized therapy techniques. The association between the therapeutic relationship and client outcome is strongest when measured by client ratings of both constructs. Some therapists are better than others at contributing to positive client outcome. Clients characterize such therapists as more understanding and accepting, empathic, warm, and supportive. These therapists engage less often in negative behaviors such as blaming, ignoring, neglecting, rejecting, or pushing a technique-based agenda when clients are resistant (Lambert & Ogles, 2004).

DO MINDFULNESS INTERVENTIONS WITH CLINICAL TRAINEES HELP THEM RELATE POSITIVELY WITH CLIENTS?

In addition to abundant research evidence showing the relationship between facilitative conditions and client outcome there is a long history of research on methods for enhancing a trainee's ability to offer these facilitative conditions, both within and stemming from the client-centered tradition. Much of this research has focused on either supervision (Watkins, 1997) or direct training in "interpersonal skills" such as empathy (Lambert & Ogles, 1997). Research results have made it evident that empathic responding and similar skills can be quickly taught by combining instruction, modeling, practice, and feedback. This direct teaching is more effective than traditional supervision and similar unsystematic and unfocused methods for teaching such skills. Skills can be performed at high levels on demand following training but don't generalize well to routine care following training; they do not appear to be internalized by a majority of trainees. That is, training appears to increase the ability of novice therapists to be empathic, but not their inclination to use this ability in everyday practice. Research therefore suggests that "interpersonal skills" are much easier to teach than attitudes (Lambert & Ogles, 1997).

In addition, therapist attitudes characterized by warmth, unconditional positive regard or acceptance, and genuineness have proved quite difficult to teach as a skill. Training programs have either neglected these personal attitudes or relied upon personal psychotherapy, sensitivity training, and the like for their development. In this regard mindfulness training may be an extremely promising addition to clinical training because it may indeed foster attitude change (internalization) toward greater acceptance and positive regard of self and others.

Research to establish that mindfulness interventions with trainees or therapists lead to improved therapeutic relationships or outcomes for clients is a wide open field. In Chapter 1 Hick reviews the few studies that exist. Certainly changing trainee attitudes, assumptions, and beliefs through mindfulness will require more time-intensive involvement than training in interpersonal skills. The ideal amount of such training is yet to be determined. In addition, if history is any indicator, mindfulness as a method of enhancing trainee–client relationship quality may be more effective than training focused on desired training goals only when longer-term outcomes are examined—that is, when internalization of mindfulness occurs and sustains therapist behaviors of acceptance, understanding, warmth, respect, and the like across time.

WHAT ARE THE IMPLICATIONS OF RELATIONSHIP RESEARCH FOR MINDFULNESS PRACTICE?

While this volume concerns mindfulness as an approach to facilitate the therapeutic relationship, most research on mindfulness has explored it as a particular technique to teach clients. Mindfulness-based interventions are arousing considerable interest and showing promising results across a variety of disorders (Bach & Hayes, 2002; Kabat-Zinn, 1990; Ma & Teasdale, 2004; Tacon, Caldera, & Ronaghan, 2004). The broader range of mindfulness-based interventions is described in Chapter 1. To those doing research in this area, differences in the specific procedures that operationalize mindfulness are seen as important distinctions that produce different results. From the outside, such variability in methods appears more subtle than substantial. At this time not enough research has been conducted to clarify the empirical differences in outcomes that can be attributed to mindfulness as a specific technique. Unfortunately, research studies up to this point have usually focused on systematic attempts at facilitating mindfulness meditation as an adjunct to CBT, often with small total sample numbers and less than ideal control conditions. This makes it very difficult to separate the unique contribution of mindfulness as a technique from other aspects of treatment.

As use of mindfulness practices becomes more widespread, practitioners and researchers seem likely to focus attention on specific techniques and make the assumption that proper training in technique will result in effective practice—practice that maximizes client outcomes because it has been properly performed. No treatment approach is effective for everyone, and this is likely to be the case with mindfulness as well. In randomized clinical trials of specific therapies (e.g., CBT, psychodynamic) for specific disorders, about 35–40% of patients experience no benefit and a small group of patients deteriorate, perhaps 5–10% (Lambert & Ogles, 2004). In routine practice examining a wide variety of psychological treatments the usual outcomes of treatment are less impressive, with the likely number of deteriorators/nonresponders estimated to be around 40 to 70%, depending on treatment setting, disorder, and amount of psychotherapy (Hansen, Lambert, & Forman, 2002). Although evidence on mindfulness training outcomes as a technique-oriented approach to change do not yet allow for general estimates of improvement and deterioration, case studies suggest that deterioration attributed to mindfulness practices with patients does occur and needs to be attended to (Kostanski et al., 2006), especially, perhaps, in intensive training and applications in a group format.

Monitoring dynamics of the therapeutic alliance may be of special value in group treatments, where therapists might be less in touch with clients and with their own reactions. Piper (2005) studied both patient-rated alliance and therapist-rated alliance and found that, especially for patient-rated alliance, both the initial level of alliance and the linear pattern of alliance were directly and significantly related to favorable outcome. Interestingly enough for therapist-rated alliance, no significant direct relationship with outcome was found.

Given that therapists may be inattentive to the client's need for alliance, that a portion of clients are not helped, and that a minority may have a negative response to treatment, it is recommended that practitioners routinely incorporate methods of formally tracking treatment response and common factors, primarily the therapeutic alliance, at each treatment or training session. We believe that representatives of each school of psychotherapy can profit from such tracking, including mindfulness practitioners. We propose here that, especially for those clients predicted to have a poor treatment outcome, monitoring the therapeutic relationship empirically is an important way to ensure a positive client–therapist relationship.

ENHANCING MINDFULNESS PRACTICE USING TRACKING, ALERTING, AND CLINICAL SUPPORT TOOLS

Our practice suggestion begins with the application of research to mindfulness practice to enhance client outcomes. Outcome is defined conceptually as including symptoms of psychopathology, interpersonal difficulties, social role functioning, and well-being. The elements of these constructs are operationally defined in a 45-item self-report scale (Outcome Questionnaire-45; Lambert, Morton, et al., 2004) that can be administered on a session-by-session basis throughout the course of an intervention. The scale was constructed and validated with particular attention to the inclusion of items that remain constant over time if a person goes untreated but demonstrates positive change with increasing sessions of psychotherapy.

Following the progress of thousands of clients over the course of treatment led to the generation of expected recovery curves and the determination of the amount of deviation from expected recovery that is predictive of a poor outcome. From this information, an empirically derived signal-alarm system for providing ongoing feedback to therapists (with particular emphasis on providing feedback about potential treatment failure) was developed and its predictive accuracy was tested and supported (Finch, Lambert, & Schaalje, 2001; Hannon et al., 2005; Lambert, Whipple, Bishop, et al., 2002). This signal-alarm system ultimately led to the creation of software (OQ-Analyst; *www.oqmeasures.com*) for providing this information to therapists and clients session by session as clients complete the measure on a weekly basis using a handheld computer with a wireless connection to the therapist's computer.

The signal-alarm system has been successfully implemented in four clinical trials that clearly demonstrate that feedback provided to therapists about impending treatment failure improves the outcome for clients at risk of having no response to treatment or a negative outcome (Hawkins, Lambert, Vermeersch, Slade, & Tuttle, 2004; Lambert et al., 2001; Lambert, Whipple, Vermeersch, et al., 2002; Whipple et al., 2003). These studies led to the development and use of Clinical Support Tools (CST) emphasizing common factors to be used with nonresponding clients (Lambert, Whipple, Harmon, et al., 2004). These tools quantify the therapeutic alliance and also assess motivation and expectancy for a positive outcome, degree of social support, maladaptive perfectionism, and recent life events. The recognition of potential treatment failure (signal-alarm) and the relationship ratings provide therapists with an indication that alliance ruptures and related problems may be hindering progress (Harmon et al., 2007). The CST provides suggestions for interventions and helps therapists become more responsive to clients when they receive a signal from the software output that the client is not progressing.

These methods may be a valuable complement to mindfulness practices in which subjective observation of self-process on the part of the client and trainee is centrally valued. Psychological assessments of ongoing functioning can be considered as a "lab test" or as the quantification of psychological "vital signs" that allow others to observe states of being. It may also provide a useful research tool for exploring the effects of mindfulness on the therapeutic relationship.

REFERENCES

American Psychological Association. (2006). Evidence-based practice in psychology. *American Psychologist, 61*(4), 271–285.

Bach, P., & Hayes, S. C. (2002). The use of acceptance and commitment therapy to prevent the rehospitalization of psychotic patients: A randomized controlled trial. *Journal of Consulting and Clinical Psychology, 70,* 1129–1139.

Castonguay, L. G., Goldfried, M. R., Wiser, S., Raue, P. J., & Hayes, A. M. (1996). Predicting the effect of cognitive therapy for depression: A study of unique and common factors. *Journal of Consulting and Clinical Psychology, 65,* 497–504.

DeRubeis, R. J., & Feeley, M. (1991). Determinants of change in cognitive therapy for depression. *Cognitive Therapy and Research, 14,* 469–482.

Elliott, R., Clark, C., & Kemeny, V. (1991, July). *Analyzing clients' post-session accounts of significant therapy events.* Paper presented at the conference of the Society for Psychotherapy Research, Lyon, France.

Finch, A. E., Lambert, M. J., & Schaalje, B. G. (2001). Psychotherapy quality control: The statistical generation of expected recovery curves for integration into an early warning system. *Clinical Psychology and Psychotherapy, 8,* 231–242.

Fonagy, P. (2006). Mechanisms of change in mentalization-based treatment of BPD. *British Journal of Clinical Psychology, 62,* 411–430.

Freud, S. (1958). On the beginning of treatment: Further recommendations on the technique of psychoanalysis. In J. Strachey (Ed. and Trans.), *Standard edition of the complete psychological works of Sigmund Freud* (Vol. 12, pp. 122–144). London: Hogarth Press. (Original work published 1913)

Gajowy, M., Marchewka, D., Sala, P., & Simon, W. (2004). [Analysis of drop-outs from group psychotherapy in regards to patient's variables.] [*Psychotherapy*] *Psychoterapia, 2*(129), 47–55.

Gaston, L. (1990). The concept of the alliance and its role in psychotherapy: Theoretical and empirical considerations. *Psychotherapy, 27,* 143–153.

Grawe, K., Caspar, F., & Ambuhl, H. (1990). Differentielle psychotherapie-forschung: Vier therapieforman in Vergleich [Differential psychotherapy research: Four therapy format comparisons]. *Zeitschrift for Klinische Psychologie [Journal of Clinical Psychology], 19,* 287–376.

Greenson, R. R. (1965). The working alliance and the transference neurosis. *Psychoanalytic Quarterly, 34,* 155–181.

Hannan, C., Lambert, M. J., Harmon, C., Nielsen, S. L., Smart, D. W., Shimokawa, K., et al. (2005). A lab test and algorithms for identifying clients at risk for treatment failure. *Journal of Clinical Psychology: In Session, 61,* 155–163.

Hansen, N. B., Lambert, M. J., & Forman, E. V. (2002). The psychotherapy dose-response effect and its implications for treatment delivery services. *Clinical Psychology: Science and Practice, 9,* 329–343.

Harmon, S. C., Lambert, M. J., Smart, D. W., Hawkins, E. J., Nielsen, S. L., Slade, K., et al. (2007). Enhancing outcome for potential treatment failures: Therapist/client feedback and clinical support tools. *Psychotherapy Research, 17,* 379–392.

Hatcher, R. L., & Barends, A. W. (1996). Patients' view of the alliance in psychotherapy: Exploratory factor analysis of three alliance measures. *Journal of Consulting and Clinical Psychology, 64,* 1326–1336.

Hawkins, E. J., Lambert, M. J., Vermeersch, D. A., Slade, K., & Tuttle, K. (2004). The effects of providing patient progress information to therapists and patients. *Psychotherapy Research, 14*, 308–327.

Horvath, A. O., & Bedi, R. P. (2002). The alliance. In J. C. Norcross (Ed.), *Psychotherapy relationships that work: Therapist contributions and responsiveness to patients* (pp. 37–69). New York: Oxford University Press.

Horvath, A. O., & Greenberg, L. S. (1989). Development and validation of the Working Alliance Inventory. *Journal of Counseling Psychology, 36*, 223–233.

Horvath, A. O., & Greenberg, L. S. (Eds.). (1994). *The working alliance: Theory, research, practice.* New York: Wiley.

Horvath, A. O., & Luborsky, L. (1993). The role of the therapeutic alliance in psychotherapy. *Journal of Consulting and Clinical Psychology, 61*, 561–573.

Howgego, I. M., Yellowlees, P., Owen, V., Meldrum, L., & Dark, F. (2003). The therapeutic alliance: The key to effective patient outcome? A descriptive review of the evidence in community mental health case management. *Australian and New Zealand Journal of Psychiatry, 37*, 169–183.

Johnson, J., Burlingame, G., Olsen, J., Davies, D., & Gleave, R. (2006). Group climate, cohesion, alliance and empathy in group psychotherapy: Multilevel structural equation models. *Journal of Counseling Psychology, 52*(3), 310–321.

Kabat-Zinn, J. (1990). *Full catastrophe living: Using the wisdom of your body and mind to face stress.* New York: Delacorte.

Kostanski, M., Hassed, C., Gullone, E., Ciechomski, L., Chambers, R., & Allen, N. (2006). Mindfulness and mindfulness-based psychotherapy. *Psychotherapy in Australia, 12*, 10–23.

Lafferty, P., Beutler, L. E., & Crago, M. (1991). Differences between more and less effective psychotherapists: A study of select therapist variables. *Journal of Consulting and Clinical Psychology, 57*, 76–80.

Lambert, M. J., DeJulio, S. S., & Stein, D. M. (1978). Therapist interpersonal skills: Process, outcome, methodological considerations and recommendations for future research. *Psychological Bulletin, 85*, 467–489.

Lambert, M. J., Morton, J. J., Hatfield, D., Harmon, C., Hamilton, S., Reid, R. C., et al. (2004). *Administration and Scoring Manual for the Outcome Questionnaire-45.* Orem, UT: American Professional Credentialing Services.

Lambert, M. J., & Ogles, B. M. (1997). The effectiveness of psychotherapy supervision. In C. E. Watkins (Ed.), *Handbook of psychotherapy supervision* (pp. 421–446). New York: Wiley.

Lambert, M. J., & Ogles, B. M. (2004). The efficacy and effectiveness of psychotherapy. In M. J. Lambert (Ed.), *Bergin and Garfield's handbook of psychotherapy and behavior change* (5th ed., pp. 139–193). New York: Wiley.

Lambert, M. J., Whipple, J. L., Bishop, M. J., Vermeersch, D. A., Gray, G. V., & Finch, A. E. (2002). Comparison of empirically derived and rationally derived methods for identifying clients at risk for treatment failure. *Clinical Psychology and Psychotherapy, 9*, 149–164.

Lambert, M. J., Whipple, J. L., Harmon, C., Shimokawa, K., Slade, K., & Christopherson, C. (2004). *Clinical Support Tools Manual.* Provo, UT: Department of Psychology, Brigham Young University.

Lambert, M. J., Whipple, J. L., Smart, D. W., Vermeersch, D. A., Nielsen, S. L., & Hawkins, E. J. (2001). The effects of providing therapists with feedback on client progress during psychotherapy: Are outcomes enhanced? *Psychotherapy Research, 11*, 49–68.

Lambert, M. J., Whipple, J. L., Vermeersch, D. A., Smart, D. W., Hawkins, E. J., Nielsen, S.

L., et al. (2002). Enhancing psychotherapy outcomes via providing feedback on client progress: A replication. *Clinical Psychology and Psychotherapy, 9,* 91–103.

Lazarus, A. A. (1971). *Behavior therapy and beyond.* New York: McGraw-Hill.

Lorr, M. (1965). Client perceptions of therapists. *Journal of Consulting Psychology, 29,* 146–149.

Luborsky, L. B. (1994). Therapeutic alliances as predictors of psychotherapy outcomes: Factors explaining the predictive success. In A. O. Horvath & L. S. Greenberg (Eds.), *The working alliance: Theory, research, and practice* (pp. 38–50). New York: Wiley.

Luborsky, L., McClellan, A. T., Woody, G. E., O'Brien, C. P., & Auerbach, A. (1985). Therapist success and its determinants. *Archives of General Psychiatry, 42,* 602–611.

Ma, S. H., & Teasdale, J. D. (2004). Mindfulness-based cognitive therapy depression: Replication and exploration of differential relapse prevention effects. *Journal of Consulting and Clinical Psychology, 72,* 31–40.

Mamodhoussen, S. (2005). Impact of marital and psychological distress on therapeutic alliance in couples undergoing couple therapy. *Journal of Marital and Family Therapy, 31*(2), 159–169.

Martin, D. J., Garske, J. P., & Davis, M. K. (2000). Relation of therapeutic alliance with outcome and other variables: A meta-analytic review. *Journal of Consulting and Clinical Psychology, 68,* 438–450.

McGuire-Snieckus, R. (2007). A new scale to assess the therapeutic relationship in community mental health care: STAR. *Psychological Medicine, 37,* 85–95.

Meissner, W. W. (2006). The therapeutic alliance—A proteus in disguise. *Psychotherapy: Theory, Research, Training, and Practice, 43,* 264–270.

Miller, W. R., Taylor, C. A., & West J. C. (1980). Focused versus broad-spectrum behavior therapy for problem drinkers. *Journal of Consulting and Clinical Psychology, 48,* 590–601.

Murphy, P. M., Cramer, D., & Lillie, F. J. (1984). The relationship between curative factors perceived by patients in their psychotherapy and treatment outcome: An exploratory study. *British Journal of Medical Psychology, 57,* 187–192.

Okiishi, J. C., Lambert, M. J., Eggett, D., Nielsen, S. L., Dayton, D., & Vermeersch, D. A. (2006). An analysis of therapist treatment effects: Toward providing feedback to individual therapists on their patients' psychotherapy outcome. *Journal of Clinical Psychology, 62,* 1157–1172.

Parloff, M., Waskow, I. E., & Wolfe, B. E. (1978). Research on therapist variables in relation to process and outcome. In A. E. Bergin & S. L. Garfield (Eds.), *Handbook of psychotherapy and behavior change* (2nd ed., pp. 233–282). New York: Wiley.

Piper, W. E. (2005). Level of alliance, pattern of alliance, and outcome in short-term group therapy. *International Journal of Group Psychotherapy, 55,* 527–550.

Ponsi, M. (2000). Therapeutic alliance and collaborative interactions. *International Journal of Psycho-Analysis, 81*(4), 687–704.

Ricks, D. F. (1974). Supershrink: Methods of a therapist judged successful on the basis of adult outcomes of adolescent patients. In D. F. Ricks, M. Roff, & A. Thomas (Eds.), *Life history research in psychopathology* (pp. 288–308). Minneapolis: University of Minnesota Press.

Rogers, C. R. (1957). The necessary and sufficient conditions of therapeutic personality change. *Journal of Consulting Psychology, 22,* 95–103.

Safran, J. D., & Wallner, L. K. (1991). The relative predictive validity of two therapeutic alliance measures in cognitive therapy. *Psychological Assessment: A Journal of Consulting and Clinical Psychology, 3,* 188–195.

Strupp, H. H., Fox, R. E., & Lessler, K. (1969). *Patients view their psychotherapy.* Baltimore: Johns Hopkins Press.

Tacon, A. M., Caldera, Y. M., & Ronaghan, C. (2004). Mindfulness-based stress reduction in women with breast cancer. *Families, Systems & Health, 22,* 193–203.

Thorne, B. (1992). *Carl Rogers.* Newbury Park, CA: Sage.

Truax, C. B. (1971). Effectiveness of counselor and counselor aids: A rejoinder. *Journal of Counseling Psychology, 18,* 365–367.

Van der Feltz-Cornelis, C. M. (2004). A patient–doctor relationship questionnaire (PDRQ-9) in primary care: Development and psychometric evaluation. *General Hospital Psychiatry, 26*(2), 115–120.

Wampold, B. E. (2001). *The great psychotherapy debate: Models, methods, and findings.* Mahwah, NJ: Erlbaum.

Watkins, C. E. (Ed.). (1997). *Handbook of psychotherapy supervision.* New York: Wiley.

Whipple, J. L., Lambert, M. J., Vermeersch, D. A., Smart, D. W., Nielsen, S. L., & Hawkins, E. J. (2003). Improving the effects of psychotherapy: The use of early identification of treatment failure and problem-solving strategies in routine practice. *Journal of Counseling Psychology, 58,* 59–68.

// THERAPEUTIC PRESENCE

While mindfulness is implicit in many philosophical and spiritual traditions, Buddhist tradition has perhaps developed it most fully and explicitly. In Buddhist tradition, mindfulness with regard to others can be described through the teaching of the *brahmaviharas*: love, compassion, joy, and equanimity. Here Thomas Bien offers insight into these practices as a way to understand the kind of presence that is truly therapeutic.

Is it ever really possible to understand another person? When we think of ourselves in relation to other selves, do we even know what we mean by "self"? Paul Fulton and Russell Walsh challenge our easy assumptions in these areas. We may often remark, "Don't take it personally," but normally we have a very circumscribed view about what things should be understood in a nonpersonal way. Fulton examines our Western assumption of the reality of self in light of the seminal Buddhist insight of no self and shows how this insight can change the way we understand the relationship between therapists and clients. Walsh, looking at the therapeutic relationship not only from a mindfulness perspective but also from the perspective of humanistic psychology, phenomenology, and hermeneutics, teaches us to be cautious about the genial assumption that we really understand another person, or that we know what we mean when we talk about being "empathic." Often such easy assurance is a barrier to the circular process of checking and rechecking our assumptions that is key to the openness and not-knowing that facilitate a rich therapeutic relationship.

3 The Four Immeasurable Minds

Preparing to Be Present in Psychotherapy

THOMAS BIEN

Your career is the career of enlightenment, of love.
—THICH NHAT HANH (1999, p. 169)

A friend related that he set out to live mindfully one day, but his efforts lasted all of 30 seconds before he gave up in frustration. Another friend commented that she liked my books about mindfulness but found it difficult to put them into practice.

If we become frustrated in trying to practice mindfulness and find ourselves giving up, it may be because it sounds simple, and we therefore expect it to be easy. We can readily understand that it would be helpful to live with full, accepting, nonjudgmental awareness of moment-by-moment experience. But when we actually try to put this simple idea into practice, it can seem daunting.

Running provides a useful analogy. Like running, mindfulness is a simple process: take this step, then this one, then this one. But one should not expect to be able to go out the first time and run a marathon. Training, practice, and persistence are required. A gentle, sustained effort is more likely to be helpful than sudden and inconsistent bursts of strained activity.

With both running and mindfulness, there can be a nearly immediate reward if one does not push too hard or overtrain. If you run just enough and not too much, even on the first time out, you can enjoy the feeling of pleasant relaxation and mild fatigue that follows exercise. Also, if you are patient and gently persistent, in a relatively short period there can be a sense of progress. Whereas at first you could only jog a few hundred yards, gradually you can come to run a half mile, then a mile, then several miles. At this point you feel encouraged, and a marathon begins to seem possible.

Similarly, with mindfulness training, it is possible to experience some relief right away. The first time you practice mindful breathing, you may be able to experience some pleasure as you follow the movements and sensations of breathing in and out. Gradually, over time, your lapses in awareness become shorter and your periods of present-centeredness grow longer. And one day, what seemed impossible in the first 30 seconds of effort becomes possible.

LEARNING TO BE A THERAPIST

The skills of a good therapist are also deceptively simple to explain but not easy to practice. For many therapists in training, the first experience with a client can be anxiety provoking. They have already acquired a knowledge base. They have a sense of what they are supposed to do. But knowing what to do and being able to do it are two quite different things—as my friends discovered when they set about living mindfully.

Fundamental to the art of the therapist is the capacity to listen in a skillful way, a way that avoids a lot of judgment, that is accepting and receptive—a way that demonstrates to the client that one is more intent on understanding than on evaluating, diagnosing, or fixing. Most schools of psychotherapy have developed a language to describe this kind of listening. In the psychoanalytic tradition, for example, the analyst is encouraged to listen to the free flowing disclosures of the analysand with an uncritical, nonjudgmental, and benign curiosity (Arlow, 1989). With the advent of Heinz Kohut's self psychology (1971), the principle of therapeutic empathy became central in psychoanalytic psychology. Kohut insisted that a remote, "experience distant" analyst was not helpful, but rather that analysts need to understand their clients in an "experience near" way.

In the family systems area, psychiatrist Murray Bowen (1978) made a related discovery. Studying people with schizophrenia and their families, Bowen found that when his research team tried to *change* these families by treating them in some way, nothing seemed to help. But when, instead, they began to study these families in order to simply *understand* what was going on, improvement seemed to follow of itself.

Humanistic psychologists have made parallel observations. Fritz Perls, originator of the Gestalt school of psychotherapy and scarcely nondirective in his therapeutic approach, noted, "Now any therapist who wants to be *helpful* is doomed right from the beginning" (Perls, 1959, p. 39). And noted humanistic psychologist Abraham Maslow presses the point vigorously:

> To the extent that we try to master the environment or be effective with it, to that extent do we cut the possibility of full, objective, detached, non-interfering cognition. Only if we let it be can we perceive fully. Again, to cite psychotherapeutic experience, the more eager we are to make a diagnosis and a plan of action, the *less* helpful do we become. The more eager we are to cure, the longer it takes. Every psychiatric researcher has to learn not to *try* to cure, *not* to be impatient. In this and in many other situations, to give in is to overcome, to be humble is to succeed. (1968, p. 184)

Perhaps the classic expression of this idea is found in Carl Rogers's (1957) seminal article on the necessary and sufficient conditions of therapeutic change. Of the six conditions of change listed in the article, three concern therapist variables. First, the therapist is *congruent* or *integrated* in the context of the relationship. This means the therapist is aware of his or her own experiencing in the context of the therapy process, even if these experiences are not what one would ideally expect of a therapist, such as feeling bored or impatient. For our purposes, we might say therapists are to be *mindful* of what they are actually feeling even when they think they should feel otherwise. Second, the therapist experiences *unconditional positive regard* for the patient. Rogers clarifies that the term *unconditional*, as he intended it, does not necessarily imply absolute, but means that the therapist harbors no *conditions* that the client has to achieve in order for the therapist to prize the client. That is, the therapist does not harbor a reservation such as "I will value this client only if he or she acts in such and such a way." Third, the therapist has an accurate, *empathic* understanding of the client's internal frame of reference and tries to communicate this experience to the client.

There is empirical support for the notion that empathy is related to positive therapeutic outcome. This literature was reviewed more extensively by Michael Lambert and Witold Simon in Chapter 2, but I will briefly cite a few examples. At the University of New Mexico, where I trained, Miller, Taylor, and West (1980) found that therapists who ranked high on empathy also ranked high on therapeutic outcome. Therapist empathy was in fact the best overall predictor of outcome, correlating an impressive .82 with treatment outcome. Needless to say, correlations of that size are highly unusual in social science. It was also surprising since this was an intervention for alcoholism, a problem that, especially at that time, was thought to require a more aggressive approach smashing through a personality structure characterized by overuse of primitive defense mechanisms such as denial. My own research (Bien, Miller, & Boroughs, 1993) found that an empathic approach to inpatients with severe alcoholism improved treatment outcome when added at random to the treatment already afforded by the hospital. Other examples are not hard to find (Burns & Nolen-Hoeksema, 1991; Miller & Sovereign, 1989; Patterson & Forgatch, 1985; Vaillant, 1994; Valle, 1981).

What we have, then, in these and other sources, are important hints about the kind of attitude or mental set that is helpful in a therapist: "experience near," empathic, open and receptive, more focused on understanding than on diagnosing or on technique. These and other ways of describing the way that the ideal therapist is present with a client are contained in the term *mindfulness*. Mindfulness is a quality of nonjudgmental, open, accepting awareness in the here and now (among many sources, Bien, 2006; Bien & Bien, 2002, 2003; see also Hick, Chapter 1, this volume). Subjectively, it represents an accepting attitude toward inner experience—toward thoughts, feelings, and sensations. In an interpersonal context, it is the embodiment of the kind of attitude described above, warm and accepting, kindly and compassionate without being possessive and without conditions that the client must meet to merit such attention. Psychotherapeutic approaches based on mindfulness have been growing in both popularity and in empirical support (e.g., Baer, 2006; Germer, Siegel, & Fulton, 2005; Hayes, Strosahl, & Wilson, 1999; Linehan, 1993; and Segal, Williams, & Teasdale, 2002). Whether mindfulness is something that therapists can teach without practicing it themselves is a matter of debate. Hayes et al. (1999) have approached the problem primarily as a set of techniques to teach clients, while Segal et al. (2002) discovered that they could not teach this approach without becoming practitioners of it themselves.

Elsewhere (Bien, 2006) I have outlined a different approach, suggesting that the main use of mindfulness may lie in fostering a certain kind of presence in the therapist, more than viewing mindfulness as a therapeutic technique or a set of skills one teaches clients. There I describe mindful therapy as the capacity of the therapist to produce true presence and deep listening. The advantage of this approach is that it may, for one thing, help therapists be more at ease in their work, while offering flexibility about the extent to which mindfulness is taught directly to clients. Such flexibility is important in that not all clients are open to the same kinds of techniques, and some in fact may have religious or other objections to practicing mindfulness. Numerous empirical questions involved here await investigation, but therapists need not wait for these to explore for themselves whether practicing mindfulness provides a sense of greater ease and effectiveness in their work, whatever their therapeutic orientation.

The approach I have described is explicitly rooted in Buddhist teaching, not as a religion or dogma, but as a set of practices designed to evoke a new way of perceiving. Some psychologists have been reluctant to approach mindfulness from a too explicitly Buddhist point of view. This may be because, in the West, religions are viewed as in competition with one another and tend more toward active proselytizing. It is quite possible, however, to view Buddhism as itself a wise, ancient, practical psychology rather than a religion in our usual sense of the word, and in fact, many practitioners of Buddhism approach it in exactly this kind of spirit. Indeed, it is possible to consider oneself a Buddhist without having any particular beliefs or dogmas resembling religious ones (Batchelor, 1997). In this sense, we can enrich our understanding of mindfulness through acquaintance with its Buddhist roots, without fear of adopting a religion that may threaten any particular weltanschauung—whether our own or our clients'.

MENTAL TRAINING

While traditional training for psychotherapists involves gaining a knowledge base and a set of techniques, little attention has been paid to the cultivation of the kind of attitude that might facilitate the therapeutic relationship and therapeutic outcome. Buddhism, on the other hand, is a 2,500-year-old tradition that, through the centuries, has been devoted to mental training. The Sanskrit word *dhyana*, often translated as meditation, is actually better understood more broadly as mental training. Mindfulness is one form of such mental training. In many ways, it is in fact the central form of mental training in Buddhism (Nhat Hanh, 1998).

To appreciate the value of mindfulness, it can help to understand the metaphysical background of this practice. Ancient India offers an image of the nature of the universe in the net of the god Indra. Indra's net holds a jewel at each intersection, with each jewel simultaneously reflecting all the others. In other words, this is a picture of a holographic universe, in which each part contains all the other parts. This is a universe that is nondualistic, that cannot, ultimately, be separated into bits. Because of this, in Buddhist thinking, to touch one time deeply is to touch all times, and to touch one thing deeply is to touch all things. Buddhist teaching functions this way as well, so that the various practices are not ultimately seen as separate but deeply interrelated. In his first teaching, the Buddha described eight limbs or aspects of practice, known as the noble eightfold path. Without enumerating all of them here, two of these aspects are right speech and right mindfulness. Right speech is speech that is true and kind, avoids exaggeration, and does not spread rumors. But right speech cannot ultimately be separated from right mindfulness. It will not be possible to practice right speech unless one is mindful. And if you are mindful, you will end up speaking in this way.

We sometimes try to separate out the various components of good therapy: what kinds of statements therapists make, what sorts of questions to ask, how to ask them, tone of voice, reflection, validation, therapeutic boundaries, when and how to offer approaches to change, what approaches to offer, and more. To teach, one must inevitably try to break expert therapist behavior into such components. It is unavoidable. Nonetheless, all of these ways of acting are rooted in a certain kind of presence—a presence that involves an intention to listen in a certain way, to avoid causing harm, and to be fully present. Just as the Buddha talked about right speech, however, he also talked about mindfulness as the kind of awareness that underlies all these other practices. Given the importance of the common factors in therapy, it might make sense to try to teach the kind of *attitude* that is therapeutic, the stance, if you will, of the therapist. And just as mindfulness encompasses the other practices in Buddhism, mindfulness can be a useful way to think about the underlying attitude of the therapist, encompassing and underlying everything the therapist does.

A Buddhist teaching that relates directly to mindfulness in an interpersonal context is the teaching of the Four Immeasurable Minds, or *brahmaviharas*[1] (Nhat Hanh, 1997, 1998). *Brahma* is a Sanskrit word for God, and a *vihara* is an abode or dwelling place. To practice the Four Immeasurable Minds is, in other words, to dwell in the divine realm, the realm some Buddhists call the Pure Land of the Buddha. To describe this practice in such terms signifies high regard for its transformative value, engendering a deep change in perception such that the ordinary world of sorrow and delusion (samsara) reveals itself as the realm of bliss (nirvana).

The Four Immeasurable Minds are love (in Pali, *metta*, in Sanskrit, *maitri*), compassion (*karuna* in both languages), joy (*mudita*), and equanimity (*upekkha* in Pali, *upeksha* in Sanskrit). While these terms may seem soft and poetic to scientific ears, they actually have precise meanings and involve practices and mental training rather than referring solely to emotional states. Love, in this context, means the capacity to offer joy and happiness (Nhat Hanh, 1998). Note that this does not mean simply the *intention* to offer joy and happiness. The intention may be the beginning, but it is insufficient. It is also the *capacity* to offer joy and happiness, meaning that one has the requisite skill to offer this. *Metta* is sometimes translated as "lovingkindness" to differentiate it from romantic love, which from a Buddhist point of view is more of an attachment than it is true *metta*. The Sanskrit word *maitri* comes from the same stem as the word for friendship, which provides another clue about what is meant: it is the kind of love one might have for a friend.

Compassion here is the capacity to offer relief from suffering (Nhat Hanh, 1998). Once again, this involves skill as well as intention. Offering compassion in this sense is not just about having a feeling of sadness regarding the client's difficulties. In fact, compassion is not a great translation of the Buddhist idea, since our word *compassion* (*com* [with] + *passio* [to suffer]) implies that one suffers with the other person. In the Buddhist practice of *karuna*, however, it is not necessary to feel sadness for the other person to the point of suffering on their behalf, as though this somehow did the other person good. In this sense it is somewhat like the work of a physician who offers a helpful prescription or other treatment. A caring physician may care deeply about a patient but need not actually suffer with the patient to bring healing.

To offer love, to offer joy and happiness, there must be understanding. To give a recording of rap music to someone who finds such music unpleasant is not *metta*. Such an action lacks a deep understanding of the person and what brings that person happiness. Such a gift is unskillful at best.

Similarly, to offer a client joy and happiness, the therapist must have a clear and deep perception of who that person is, and how things stand in the moment-by-moment, shifting process of therapy. Out of this perception, a therapist will not just woodenly offer any technique, but will offer what is needed for this person in this situation. In some cases, perhaps in many cases, that will be helpful. For example, more often than we imagine, reflective listening is the best way to offer happiness and relieve suffering. Too frequently we imagine we have to do something, make an interpretation or offer an exercise or a plan of action, when in reality our presence and listening would help more. However, there are also times when it is unempathic and unkind to withhold concrete information or advice. The attuned therapist is not rigid or doctrinaire about such matters and does not confuse attitude with technique, but flows with the changing currents of the therapeutic encounter.

The third immeasurable mind is joy. *Mudita* is sometimes translated as "sympathetic joy" to connect it to the good fortune of others. But in the context of the nondualistic point of view described above with the metaphor of the net of Indra, such a description is overly restrictive (Nhat Hanh, 1997). In the interpenetrating, profoundly interconnected world of noself, there is no need to discriminate between one's own joy and the joy of another person. We may usefully compensate for the natural tendency to focus on our own experiences by making a special effort to be aware of the joys of others, but it is important for us to be in touch with our own joy as well.

In a therapy context, joy is an important element, though perhaps not one that is explicitly described in many books about therapy. Joy here means first of all that at times there can be a lightness in the therapeutic encounter. While care obviously needs to be taken that one is not out of harmony with the internal state of the client, there can be jokes, stories, and laughter in psychotherapy, even when talking about serious and sad things. Joy is also about finding a way to *enjoy* the company of our clients. In some sessions therapists and clients can discuss incredibly painful losses and difficulties but still be able to laugh together and enjoy a moment of lightness before returning to a more somber mood. One therapist I heard about prevented a suicide in a phone conversation by telling knock-knock jokes and getting the client to laugh. The story may be apocryphal, and, since it involves what might appear a nonempathic response to the client's distress, I would not recommend it as a general technique. Still, it makes the point that there is a place for laughter and humor. By such means, we offer the perspective that, as there are sad elements in humor and laughter, so there also can be bright elements in dark times. We do not need to be trapped in a given mood or emotional atmosphere. In fact, we may honor it more by not being totally engulfed in it.

While therapists may be prepared to step into their clients' worlds to understand their sorrows and difficulties, we less often consider it our work to enter deeply into their joys and good fortune. Yet this is just as important. Without the energy of joy, it is difficult to withstand the withering attacks of our problems in living. Joy is what makes it possible for us to be in contact with sorrow and not be submerged in it. If we are to be therapeutic mirrors who reflect back to our clients an understanding of their difficulties, then we can also be mirrors who reflect back their joys, letting these touch us just as fully and just as deeply. A joy shared is multiplied, and may increase a client's resilience in the face of painful difficulties.

If we are to avoid a dualistic split between our own joy and the joy of others, then joy also implies that we as therapists must be in touch with that which provides joy in our own lives. Without joy, we may find ourselves becoming too distant from a client's pain, unable to bear it because there is so much sorrow in our own lives. It is the difference between a plant that has been well watered the day before and is then exposed to the hot sun, and one that has received no water. Without joy, we wilt.

Equanimity, the fourth immeasurable mind, is also a crucial element. Equanimity means evenness, the capacity to accept whatever comes undisturbed. It is not indifference. It doesn't entail being unfeeling, but means not getting lost in the feeling, in the endless dramatizing and storytelling that fuses us with feelings, but instead seeing our sadness as just sadness with nothing extra added, our anger as just anger, even our happiness and peace as just happiness and peace, all of which arises from moment to moment and then passes away. Rogers (1957) made a similar point when he wrote that empathy is experiencing the client's world *as if* it were one's own, but without ever losing this "as if" quality. Without the "as if," we become fused with our experience. We become caught in it, contained rather than containing. Unless there is equanimity in our love and compassion, we will suffer in our work, and also ultimately be less effective. We as therapists require a clear, keen sense that we cannot make our clients' choices for them, nor can we alter the facts of the natural world. We know that these difficulties are the client's difficulties and resist overidentifying with them. Just as, in practicing mindfulness of thinking, we know that our thoughts are just thoughts, that we are larger than the thoughts, so equanimity teaches us to enter into our clients' painful experience without getting lost or overwhelmed. In this sense, it becomes vital to understand that *karuna* is not "compassion" in the sense of literally suffering with the client.

You may have had the experience of discussing a personal difficulty with a friend who overidentifies with your distress so that the friend becomes as distressed and as troubled as you are. Though sometimes people can even take pride in this kind of "compassion," thinking it means that they are heroically sensitive to the pain of other people, it is not helpful. Some Buddhists call this "idiot compassion," like offering ice cream to a diabetic. Instead of one distressed person, now there are two. Nothing good is likely to come out of such a situation. Two drowning people clutching at each other both go under. What is needed is one person with both feet clearly planted on terra firma who can then extend a pole to the drowning person.

These four elements work concertedly rather than independently. If our love and compassion do not have equanimity in them, they may be something other than love and compassion. They may be manipulation. They may be an effort to build up an account of favors to draw on in the future. They may be an attempt to instill guilt. Our love and compassion are not love and compassion unless they allow the other person space and freedom, including the freedom to make bad choices. Love and compassion without equanimity will have an uncomfortable quality, an emotional "stickiness" that leaves one suspicious of the caregiver's true intention.

The effect is similar if one's love and compassion are lacking in joy. If you can only empathize with someone's sorrows, without also appreciating their joys, your compassion may not be true compassion. Perhaps your compassion is more a matter of helping yourself to feel good by offering the supportive shoulder, building yourself up as the strong person in the context of another's distress. Without joy, you may actually leave a person more stuck in their grief and sadness than they were before.

The interconnection between joy and equanimity is expressed well in the saying of Buddhist teacher Long Chen Pa: "Since everything is none other than exactly the way it is, one may well just break out in laughter" (cited in Kornfield, 2000). Acknowledging the truth and accepting it fully, including the difficulties of our lives, need not result in nihilism or despair, but can result in the joy that comes when we stop struggling against the nature of things.

If you are truly mindful of another person, your mindfulness contains love, compassion, joy, and equanimity. If any one of these elements is lacking, then all are lacking. If any one of these elements is lacking, then mindfulness itself is not present.

BENEFITS OF LOVE AND COMPASSION

While equanimity must be present in practicing the *brahmaviharas*, lest our love and compassion have a sticky, manipulative quality, the practices of love and compassion also benefit the practitioner. In this sense, there is an element of enlightened egoism in this practice. Looking deeply, looking at this in the context of nondualism, we cannot ultimately separate our own well-being from that of another. The greatest gift we give to others is first of all to be a happy person. By doing things that foster our own happiness, we make it possible to offer happiness to others. Without happiness in ourselves, we are powerless to do so. Conversely, if we are unhappy, and live in a way that fosters unhappiness, we become a burden to others. Our unhappiness spreads from us like a contagion. In Buddhist teaching, this is the insight of what is called the second dharma seal, the insight of non-self or interbeing (Nhat Hanh, 1998, pp. 124–126; Bien, 2006, pp. 150–158; see also Marlatt et al., Chapter 7, this volume). Thus, I often tell clients their happiness is job one.

In the sutras, the Buddha teaches that one who practices *metta* will receive the following benefits: (1) sleeping well, (2) waking up feeling well and light of heart, (3) having no unpleasant dreams, (4) being liked by and at ease with others, especially children, (5) being dear to animals, (6) being supported and protected by gods and goddesses, (7) protection from fire, poison, and sword, (8) being able to attain meditative concentration easily, (9) having one's face become bright and clear, (10) mental clarity at the time of death, and (11) being reborn in the Brahma heaven (Nhat Hanh, 1997). Whatever one makes of such traditional language, and however one chooses to interpret it, one can clearly see that the Buddha thought this was an important and highly beneficial practice.

In an often reported experiment, students watching a film of Mother Teresa working with the poor in Calcutta showed an increase in levels of s-IgA in their saliva, indicating improved immune functioning, regardless of whether they approved or disapproved of Mother Teresa and her work (McClelland, 1986).

An exploration at the University of Wisconsin (reported in Barasch, 2005) demonstrated some tantalizing neurological findings regarding love and compassion. A Buddhist monk named Matthieu Ricard (referred to as Lama Öser) was monitored on a functional MRI while he practiced lovingkindness meditation. This is how he described what he was doing: "Let there be only compassion and love in the mind for all beings—friends and loved ones, strangers and enemies alike. It's compassion with no agenda, that excludes no one. You generate this quality of loving, and let it soak the mind." The MRI revealed a dramatic increase in activation of the left middle frontal gyrus, an area associated with joy and enthusiasm. Ricard was also found to be two standard deviations above the norm on a task involving the perception of rapid changes in facial expressions of emotion, a capacity that correlates with empathy. It is always possible, of course, that single-subject investigations such as this measure some special capacity of the individual rather than something generalizable to others. Yet Ricard insists that his capacity for this sort of meditation was not particularly advanced relative to other practitioners.

CULTIVATING LOVE, COMPASSION, JOY, AND EQUANIMITY

These qualities, then, may be helpful to a therapist in many ways. One way they can help is by lightening the load. I began the first chapter of *Mindful Therapy* (Bien, 2006) with the sentence "Therapy is not easy work." I did this very intentionally, out of a Buddhist understanding that it is important to speak the truth of our situation without sugarcoating it. If we can say that therapy can be very rewarding work, that it is wonderful to see how some clients grow and change, we should say that it is also very difficult. We sit with people who are very distressed, and not always pleasant. Distressed people sometimes look for someone to blame for their distress, creating the risk that we who try to be present with them in those problems will become a ready target.

One might be tempted to lighten the burden of the work through indifference. In my perception, however, this is ineffective. It is ineffective because indifference is not a therapeutic stance. But I think it also doesn't work because when we become indifferent, our clients' difficulties become an irritation. But if we cultivate equanimous compassion, we become large enough to take in the client's distress without suffering because of it ourselves. Because of equanimity, we see clearly that we cannot control the 40% of the variance accounted for by factors outside of therapy (Lambert, 1992). Deep acknowledgment and acceptance of this reality offer the possibility of both greater peace and an enhanced ability to be present.

It may also make us more effective. By being mindful, by practicing kindness, compassion, joy, and equanimity, we may enhance our capacity to be concerned and present without overidentification—the very qualities Rogers (1957) and Kohut (1971) and Maslow (1968) and so many others have talked about, and the very qualities that account for so much of the variance (30% for "common factors" vs. 15% for "techniques") described by Lambert (1992). Even this may underestimate the importance of these factors, since therapy ultimately is a lived inter-action, an ongoing stream of listening and responding that cannot be separated from the whole, even if it is heuristically useful to do so. For this reason, technique delivered in a well-timed, empathic fashion may be far more helpful than technique outside of such a context.

But then, if mindfulness as described here—kindness and compas-sion, joy and equanimity—can be so helpful, how then can an individ-ual therapist cultivate these qualities? Traditional contemplative exer-cises from Buddhism and other traditions suggest some possibilities.

In the Christian contemplative tradition, there is a practice known as *lectio divina*. This practice arises from the notion that the study of scriptural texts should lead naturally into contemplation. As one stud-ies the scripture, one can take a word or phrase that one finds particu-larly striking and simply hold it in one's awareness for a time. Similarly, one can learn to simply dwell with words like *love, kindness, joy, peace,* or *letting go* as one breathes gently in and out. What is essential in this kind of practice is to do it in such a way that one stays in contact with the meaning of the words, rather than repeating them mechanically.

Such practices make sense in the context of Buddhist psychology. In this psychology (the *Abhidharma*), we have many *bija*, or seeds, which represent potential psychological states (Nhat Hanh, 2001). These states involve both positive and negative potentials, such as the potential for mindfulness or kindness, on the one hand, or anger and depression on the other. One seeks to water the positive seeds so that they grow stronger, while learning to embrace the negative seeds with mindfulness so that their potential is diminished. In such practices, as with all mindfulness-based practices, gentleness and acceptance are re-quired, rather than forcing. If one pushes too hard, there can be a back-lash, a rebound of negative emotional states. For example, if one pushes the seed of joy too hard, one may end up later feeling depressed or sad. It is helpful to remember that, from a Buddhist point of view, watering seeds of love and joy lines us up[2] with reality, so that we are in harmony with no-self (*anatta*), or interbeing—with the way things really are. Practicing gently means, for example, that if we dwell with the word *love,* but experience anger coming up instead, then we embrace the an-ger with our mindfulness. Mental training is never a matter of forcing, but rather of opening to reality

In Buddhist practice there is a long-established tradition of *metta* meditation by which one seeks to cultivate the mind of love. In the tra-ditional practice, one begins by cultivating kindness toward oneself, then toward people with whom one is close, then with strangers or "neutral" people, then, and more challengingly, with difficult people or enemies, then lastly with all beings. This practice resembles a series of expanding, concentric circles, with each level of practice becoming more difficult and more inclusive. At each level, one can breathe in and out and dwell with kindly intentions, such as (in the case of oneself, to begin with):

May I be happy.
May I be safe.

Beginning with oneself can be very important. If one attempts to extend kindness toward a difficult person, perhaps a colleague, family member, or patient, this may be too large a step without first generating kindness toward oneself, thereby acknowledging one's own difficult thoughts and emotions. With this as a base, one can then move on to friends, the neutral person, and so on. But the intention, in Buddhist practice, in beginning with oneself is to activate the proper feelings and attitudes, under the assumption that we can do this more easily for ourselves. For some individuals—those who do not feel good about themselves—it may be better to start with someone else whom they find easy to love. One woman I knew disliked herself but could begin quite easily by focusing on her cat. It was easy for her to love her cat. Once her heart was opened to her cat, she could then include herself and others in her kind awareness and intention.

The following exercise, "Lovingkindness Meditation for the Therapeutic Relationship," is a way of adapting this practice to your clients.

1. Before seeing clients, sit for a few moments and allow your attention to settle gently on the breath.

2. Imagine yourself as being surrounded and filled with absolute love, cradled in total acceptance, kindness, and benevolence. To make this concrete, think of a time when you felt deeply loved and accepted, or imagine yourself in the presence of an all-loving being, a Buddha or a Christ, or whatever image might help elicit these feelings.

3. As you continue feeling loved and accepted, gently hold the following intentions for yourself:

May I be happy.
May I be peaceful.
May I have abundance.
May I be safe.

May I have ease of well-being.
May I be free of negative emotions.

4. Envision yourself as capable not only of receiving but also of spreading this feeling of love and acceptance. Feel the presence of each person you are scheduled to see that day, evoking a global, felt sense of who they are, what their difficulties are, and what is positive about them. You might begin with those it is easy for you to feel kindly toward, and gradually expand to include those who are more difficult. Imagine yourself sitting with them, relaxed, open, and at ease, intent on understanding, letting what you say and do flow naturally from this awareness.

5. Gently hold the intentions above for your clients: "May he be happy. May she be peaceful," and so on.

6. End by enjoying a few mindful breaths.

The exact nature and wording of the intentions can vary, and one can freely invent new ones, perhaps ones that grow out of a particular life context. In fact, inventing one's own phrases may at times be especially helpful in that the words which come out of one's own consciousness and experience may be more vivid and help one stay in touch with their meaning without having them degenerate into empty sounds.

ON-THE-SPOT PRACTICE

Whenever we encounter some difficulty, whenever we find ourselves in a difficult emotional state, full of sadness, anger, or worry, the temptation is to fall deeper into ourselves, feeling more isolated and disconnected. It is helpful instead to learn, right then and there, to open one's heart to all people who are encountering similar difficulties. For example, if you are ill and the illness generates a sad or depressed state, you can imagine yourself as radiating love and compassion to all beings that are ill. If you are frustrated because a client did not accept your brilliant interpretation, you can open outward to all people who feel their efforts are not valued. I find this simple practice often brings immediate relief.

We can cultivate these attitudes the moment we greet our clients. The traditional greeting in India involves bowing and saying the word *namaste*, which means something like "I recognize the divine in you." But without bowing or using foreign words, one can simply say inwardly, "My dear friend," summoning in those words your whole felt sense of this person, her history, her struggle, and her positive qualities. Alternatively, breathe in and out and say to yourself, "I see you. I am here. I see you." When I do this, I have a sense that not only does the client become more real to me, but I am also more there, more present. Such practices help us remember that this is not just a client, but a human being like oneself, whatever the disparity in our roles.

In the midst of a session, one can always return to awareness of breathing and mindfulness, or recall a simple word such as *love* or *kindness*. Often we try so hard to be helpful as therapists, but we are struggling too much, and this in itself all but assures that we will not be helpful. Sometimes it is so easy for us to see how the person before us continues to create suffering. It is important to return to a sense of equanimity, acknowledging that one cannot change the nature of reality, or make choices for one's clients. Again, this may be done with a simple word or phrase, such as "peace," or "letting go," or, from a more explicitly Buddhist standpoint, reminding oneself to trust the wisdom or buddha nature within this person to ultimately find the way forward.

It is helpful not to rush to accomplish too many things between sessions. It need not take a lot of time to return to our breathing after a session, noting the effect the session has had on our own body and consciousness, and seeking to let it go so that we are fresh and available to the next person. This is a practice of kindness toward oneself, as well as to the next client.

A lot of research remains to be done on the effect of a therapist's meditation on psychotherapy, including both proximal, process variables, as well as distal, outcome variables. But perhaps the most important research is your own exploration of this territory, trying some of the practices above, sticking with them long enough to see an effect, perhaps creating your own methods, and exploring these effects informally. In the end, it matters little if research supports the value of having a therapist who meditates unless it also fits with your own experience.

CONCLUSION

Many therapists have written about the kind of presence that facilitates healing in clients, among them Freud, Perls, Maslow, and Rogers. There are intimations in this literature that presence may be more important than clinical technique per se. This chapter offers the Buddhist teaching of the *brahmaviharas* as way to approach both the understanding and the practice of therapeutic presence.

NOTES

1. The teaching of the *brahmaviharas* antedates Buddhism. Perhaps for this reason, some Buddhists claim that they do not represent the highest Buddhist teachings. Thich Nhat Hanh (1997, 1998) shows evidence from the Buddhist scriptures that the Buddha held these teachings in high regard.
2. *Lines us up with reality.* No-self is one of the fundamental ontological insights of Buddhism. No-self implies that reality is not best conceived as separate, isolated bits, but as highly interdependent and interpenetrating elements, such that one element implies the whole and vice versa. An apple, to use a simple example, implies the existence of the sun, for it cannot exist without solar energy converted through photosynthesis. No sun, no apple. In the same way, we are deeply interconnected with other living beings, so that their welfare and ours are inseparable. The practice of compassion is therefore like the right hand taking care of the injured left hand: it is not a morally superior action, but simply the appropriate thing to do given the underlying unity of the body. In this sense, compassionate action is in accord with what is, while action lacking in compassion is rooted in the delusion of separateness and fragmentation.

REFERENCES

Arlow, J. A. (1989). Psychoanalysis. In R. J. Corsini & D. Wedding (Eds.), *Current psychotherapies* (4th ed., pp. 19–62). Itasca, IL: F. E. Peacock.

Baer, R. (Ed.). (2006). *Mindfulness-based treatment approaches: Clinician's guide to evidence base and applications.* New York: Academic Press.

Barasch, M. I. (2005). *Field notes on the compassionate life: A search for the soul of kindness.* New York: Rodale.

Batchelor, S. (1997). *Buddhism without beliefs: A contemporary guide to awakening.* New York: Riverhead Books.

Bien, T. (2006). *Mindful therapy: A guide for therapists and helping professionals.* Boston: Wisdom.

Bien, T., & Bien, B. (2002) *Mindful recovery: A spiritual path to healing from addiction.* New York: Wiley.

Bien, T., & Bien, B. (2003). *Finding the center within: The healing way of mindfulness meditation.* Hoboken, NJ: Wiley.

Bien, T. H., Miller, W. R., & Boroughs, J. M. (1993). Motivational interviewing with alcohol outpatients. *Behavioural and Cognitive Psychotherapy, 21,* 347–356.

Bowen, M. (1978). *Family therapy in clinical practice.* New York: Jason Aronson.

Burns, D. D., & Nolen-Hoeksema, S. (1991). Coping styles, homework compliance, and the effectiveness of cognitive-behavioral therapy. *Journal of Consulting and Clinical Psychology, 59,* 305–311.

Germer, C. K., Siegel, R. D., & Fulton, P. R. (Eds.). (2005). *Mindfulness and psychotherapy.* New York: Guilford Press.

Hayes, S. C., Strosahl, K. D., & Wilson, K. G. (1999). *Acceptance and commitment therapy: An experiential approach to behavior change.* New York: Guilford Press.

Kohut, H. (1971). *The analysis of the self*. New York: International Universities Press.

Kornfield, J. (2000). *After the ecstasy the laundry: How the heart grows wise on the spiritual path*. New York: Bantam.

Lambert, M. J. (1992). Implications of outcome research for psychotherapy integration. In J. C. Norcross & M. R. Goldstein (Eds.), *Handbook of psychotherapy integration* (pp. 94–129). New York: Wiley-Interscience.

Linehan, M. M. (1993). *Cognitive-behavioral treatment of borderline personality disorder*. New York: Guilford Press.

Maslow, A. (1968). *Toward a psychology of being* (2nd ed.). New York: Van Nostrand.

McClelland, D. C. (1986). Some reflections on the two psychologies of love. *Journal of Personality, 54*(2), 344–349.

Miller, W. R., & Sovereign, R. G. (1989). The check-up: A model for early intervention in addictive behaviors. In T. Loberg, W. R. Miller, P. E. Nathan, & G. A. Marlatt (Eds.), *Addictive behaviors: Prevention and early intervention* (pp. 219–231). Amsterdam: Swets & Zeitlinger.

Miller, W. R., Taylor, C. A., & West, J. C. (1980). Focused versus broad-spectrum behavior therapy for problem drinkers. *Journal of Consulting and Clinical Psychology, 48*, 590–601.

Nhat Hanh, T. (1997). *Teachings on love*. Berkeley: Parallax Press. (See especially pp. 1–19)

Nhat Hanh, T. (1998). *The heart of the Buddha's teaching: Transforming suffering into peace, joy, and liberation*. Berkeley: Parallax Press. (See especially pp. 157–163)

Nhat Hanh, T. (1999). *Going home: Jesus and Buddha as brothers*. New York: Riverhead Books.

Nhat Hanh, T. (2001). *Transformation at the base: Fifty verses on the nature of consciousness*. Berkeley: Parallax Press.

Patterson, G. R., & Forgatch, M. S. (1985). Therapist behavior as a determinant for client noncompliance: A paradox for the behavior modifier. *Journal of Consulting and Clinical Psychology, 53*, 846–851.

Perls, F. (1959). *Gestalt therapy verbatim*. Bantam: New York.

Rogers, C. (1957). The necessary and sufficient conditions of therapeutic personality change. *Journal of Consulting Psychology, 21*(2), 95–103.

Segal, Z. V., Williams, J. M. G., & Teasdale, J. D. (2002). *Mindfulness-based cognitive therapy for depression: A new approach to preventing relapse*. New York: Guilford Press.

Vaillant, L. M. (1994). The next step in short-term dynamic psychotherapy: A clarification of objectives and techniques in an anxiety-regulating model. *Psychotherapy, 31*, 642–655.

Valle, S. K. (1981). Interpersonal functioning of alcoholism counselors and treatment outcome. *Journal of Studies on Alcohol, 42*, 783–790.

4 *Anatta*: Self, Non-Self, and the Therapist

PAUL R. FULTON

As mindfulness is adapted to psychotherapy and medicine, many concepts and practices are interpreted from Buddhism into the familiar idiom of Western psychology. The benefits to the West are many; mindfulness practices have received empirical validation from scientific study, essential elements have been distilled from peripheral or superfluous cultural accouterments, and the practices have been made available to scores of people who would ordinarily not have been exposed to them. In many instances this translation has been natural, as Western psychology has many analogues to Buddhist concepts. Where this natural overlap is lacking, the psychotherapy community has often sidestepped consideration of less accessible concepts. The idea of *anatta*, or "no-self," is one such concept, apparently esoteric, misunderstood and neglected because it has no simple referent in the lexicon of psychotherapy. However, an understanding of *anatta* (which is central to Buddhist psychology) has much to offer psychotherapy and the therapeutic relationship.

In this chapter I make a small effort to rectify that neglect, describing this elusive concept in terms that have pertinence to psychotherapy, in terms of how we understand psychotherapy's goals and limitations, and how our understanding informs the therapeutic enterprise and expands our view of the alleviation of suffering.[1]

In a brief theoretical excursion, I first explore how self is understood in the worlds of psychotherapy and mindfulness. I then explore the relevance of *anatta* for the therapist and the therapeutic relationship.

UNDERSTANDING THE SELF OF PSYCHOTHERAPY
AND THE SELF OF MINDFULNESS

Self is a universal category of experience; the capacity to distinguish oneself from another is a developmental accomplishment found cross-culturally. Anthropologist Franz Boas noted that this differentiation of self from other is codified in the pronouns of all spoken languages, distinguishing the speaker from the spoken to and the spoken of. As Beneviste said (1971, p. 225), "Consciousness of self is only possible if it is experienced by contrast." It arises in experience in the moment of taking oneself as an object, distinguishing ourselves from that which we regard as not ourselves. As such, it requires a momentary act, a *doing*. This act is accomplished symbolically and, consequently, appears to differentiate those with higher symbolic capacities (e.g., humans) from others.[2] As research methods have improved, developmental psychologists have gradually moved the age at which this nascent capacity for differentiation appears ever earlier. The differentiation of self is not a single and final accomplishment; it evolves over the course of development as our capacity for symbolic activity becomes more sophisticated.

Because this split is mediated symbolically (i.e., it is not a given, but requires some higher cortical processing), that split varies depending on the symbol systems employed; therefore, though distinguishing self from other is a universal experience, the *way* this distinction is made varies enormously across the life course, between individuals, and between cultures.[3] Who we think we are in the West cannot reliably tell us about how the Japanese or the Javanese experience themselves. Modern Westerners draw a line between self and other that is more solid, and more "narrow," than those in non-Western societies, which often regard the most meaningful boundary to exist between one's extended family or clan and those outside of it. We may all distinguish self from other, but the line between them is movable. One consequence of the role of symbols in the creation of the experience of self is that those symbols may themselves become an object of our examination. We are able to illuminate dimensions of the sense of self as a kind of common cultural experience.

Despite its universal appearance, self remains a hypothetical construct, unseen by objective measures, known only subjectively as the central organizing principle of experience. We know intuitively who we are; I am me, and me alone. But thanks to the efforts of psychological ethnography to catalog the ways self is conceived cross-culturally, we may be led to conclude that the experience of self is one that is malleable, shaped by the context in which it is found. Indeed, the experience of self cannot be distinguished from the culture's concepts used to conceive it. To have a self is to have an idea of the self, and that idea becomes inseparable from our lived, subjective experience. As Irving Hallowell pointed out (1955, p. 80), "In cross cultural perspective . . . and at the level of phenomenological description, the fact remains that human beings do function in terms of concepts of self which, in part, are culturally derived." The self-concept is a self-theory that, as noted by David Bohm (1973, p. 102), "does not remain a mere model . . . it actually becomes the self." In this way, the experience of self known in a moment of self-awareness varies with the learned symbols used to mediate this split of subject and object. This symbolic split is overdetermined, influenced by personal and collective history, gender, genetic predisposition, personality, and situational factors. This split is not unique to the West; it is formulated uniquely in every culturally indigenous psychology. For our purposes it is helpful to recognize the manner in which the self can be understood as a culturally variable product.

The Self in the West

Many social scientists see the self as originating outside the individual, or at least principally constituted in one's interaction with the social environment.[4] Western developmental psychology acknowledges the critical role of interaction with the environment in the establishment of the self. But when we step away from academic formulations—or compare our own views with those of most non-Western societies through most of known history—we discover that our collective representations and experience of self favor a different view of the individual as strangely independent and apart. In 1929 (pp. 201–202), Lucien Levy-Bruhl noted that in comparison with "primitives," "to our way of thinking, however complex an individual may be, his primordial and essential characteristic is that he shall be one person." That is, we are persons by virtue of separation, rather than by participation in the collective. Anthropologist Dorothy Lee noted that by contrast with those of other cultures (1959, p. 132).

In our commonly held unreflective view, the self is a distinct unit, something we can name and define. We know what is the self, and what is not the self: and the distinction between the two is always the same. Our own linguistic usage through the years reveals a conception of increasingly assertive, active, and even aggressive self, as well as of an increasingly delimited self.

Later, she adds:

The self is most nearly identified with consciousness and reason and will; and in our culture, reason and will power and consciousness— particularly self-consciousness—spell mastery and control. So here, too, we find the implication that the self is in control of the other.

And finally, Schweder and Bourne (1982, p. 129) wrote that in contrast to Maori culture, where an individual is valued for his or her particular deeds, in the West he or she is valued for being "a monadic replica of general humanity."

A kind of sacred personalized self is developed and the individual qua individual is seen as inviolate, a supreme value in and of itself. The "self" becomes an object of interest per se. Free to undertake projects of personal expression, personal narratives, autobiographies, diaries, mirrors, separate rooms, early separation from bed, body and breast of mother, personal space—the autonomous individual imagines the incredible, that he lives within an inviolate protected region (the extended boundaries of the self) where he is "free to choose" . . . where what he does "is his own business."

These views do not remain merely a part of our folk psychology, but find their way into our scientific view of who we are. As Vincent Crapanzano emphasized (1979, p. 3), "the degree to which our explicit psychologies are founded on the implicit psychological assumptions of our idiom." Gallimore (1981, p. 710) said it yet more directly: "It is regrettable but true that many of the concepts in social science are lay terms elevated to pseudoscientific status by repeated association with widely accepted operational definitions." Thus do we, as mental health professionals and participating members of the culture, inherit a culturally unique view of the self as autonomous. Even a casual glance reveals how this has entered into our theory (such as Margaret Mahler's emphasis on development as separation and individuation).

Just as culture helps shape our idea of how the self successfully develops into a separate, autonomous, and efficacious individual, so too does it shape how this difficult task can go awry. While many mental disorders appear universal in prevalence (in particular, major mental illnesses commonly regarded as biological, such as schizophrenia and bipolar disorders), many reflect the unique cultural stresses of their host society and are properly considered culture-bound syndromes. Given what we know about how much the sense of self is a social product, this Western, ideal developmental goal of true self-sufficiency and immutability seems unrealistic and absurd. The cultural standard of independence and autonomy is simply inconsistent with how we actually function.

Some of the "culture-bound" disorders commonly seen in the psychotherapy office arise from this tension (Lasch, 1979). For example, when we strive to become sui generis and independent, relationships become complicated challenges; how can we be intimate without abandoning ourselves? Relatedness and autonomy become somewhat opposed. Fear of dependency, or dependency itself, becomes a clinical problem to be solved. Unlike most non-Western societies, which hold less extreme notions of the separateness of self, we have an entire clinical language to describe disorders of the self: narcissistic personality disorders, fragmentation of the self (Kernberg, 1975), lack of self-cohesion (Kohut, 1977), and the ubiquitous complaint of poor self-esteem.

Just as cultures provide descriptions of how development can go wrong, they conveniently provide well matched systems of treatment and healing for those disorders. Psychotherapy is a Western contribution to Western disorders, well suited to addressing issues arising in relationship, including relationship to oneself. All methods of healing, including psychotherapy, derive much of their curative power from being embedded in the society from which they arose. It is no surprise that herbal remedies, acupuncture, and other somatic treatments are preferred to psychotherapy in Taiwan, where subjective distress is often attributed to physiological imbalances (Tseng, 1978), or that spirit worship has not caught on as a remedy in Boston.

The point of all this is that psychotherapy is originally a Western creation to address Western maladies and, for the purpose of this discussion, disorders related to self as it is understood indigenously. A cornerstone of psychotherapy is the implicit or explicit culturally congruent conception of the self. Like honeybees and flowers, psychotherapy and the self's implication in mental disease are part of a single system, depending on one another for their full meaning. And when therapy goes well, the patient is reacculturated into fuller participation in collective life through some adjustment of the self, movement toward greater selfhood, self-esteem, self-control, self-determination, efficacy, and identity.

Self in Mindfulness and Buddhist Psychology

In Buddhist psychology, the elusive developmental accomplishment of a stable sense of self is not the goal, but the point of departure for the path of mindfulness. Simply, a naive belief in oneself as a separate and enduring entity is a delusion, which gives rise to suffering. In this sense, where "ordinary human unhappiness" leaves off (Freud's famous description of the fruit of a successful psychoanalysis), Buddhist practice begins. Suffering arises from holding mistaken beliefs about who we are, or *that* we are.

In truth, Buddhist psychology claims, the separate self is an illusion, albeit persistent and compelling, and is revealed as such only with the sustained and disciplined practice of meditation. The self, Buddhists assert, is a phenomenon that arises when conditions support it and vanishes from awareness when conditions do not; there is nothing enduring, essential, or separate from the constant flux of change that is our experience. In short, it is an event, not a thing, ultimately evanescent, of no greater ontological significance than a passing thought or a physical sensation, empty of any independent or separate nature. As such, it is certainly not worthy of the devotion we heap on it.

The Pali term used for the idea of "no self" is *anatta*, often translated as "not-self."[5] This is not to connote that we don't exist in any respect—our commonsense experience cries foul at such a claim. Rather, it points to our tendency to believe that the self is more real than the evidence warrants, and to our tendency to invest it with ultimate importance, with painful results. A full account of anatta is beyond the scope of this chapter, and even if space permitted, this central Buddhist concept would likely remain one of the most difficult to grasp; even when we may be convinced of little else, we seem to know that "I am."

If the self as a separate, unchanging entity is illusory, why are we so convinced it is real? Simply, it is for failure to pay attention. Under the microscope-like lens of mindfulness, we may directly observe a number of qualities of this self experience. Close scrutiny begins to reveal how experience is momentary and constantly changing. When examining it closely, we begin to realize that the sense of continuity of things is a trick of perception, often likened to discrete frames of a movie strung together to create an illusion. In the slowed-down, up-close field of mindfulness meditation we may experience the objects of awareness *in and of themselves*, without their seeming to happen to somebody. Hearing *is*. Seeing *is*. We may have moments of full awareness without attributing it to someone behind it who is doing the seeing, hearing, thinking, and so on. We are also likely to be witness to the reappearance in awareness of self in response to our effort to control, grasp, or reject some aspect of the flow of experience. We begin to have a direct perception of self as something that we do, not something we are. Importantly, we also begin to discover the painful consequences of taking this arising of self in experience to be more real than it is.[6]

For now, it is important to note that the direct understanding of no-self is as central to Buddhist meditation practice as the Western notion of self is to psychotherapy. Above all, it is here where these practices diverge.

Narcissism East and West

In Western psychology, narcissism occupies a place as a normal developmental way station, and as a disorder when development is arrested. For Freud, self-love is a natural precursor to the capacity to love others, which only becomes a clinical problem when the overvaluation of oneself persists into later life. Much has been written in the psychoanalytic literature about the nature of pathological narcissism (notably, by Sigmund Freud, Melanie Klein, Otto Kernberg, Heinz Kohut, Henry Stack Sullivan, and Donald Winnicott) that cannot be recapped here. In broad strokes, pathological narcissism is often understood as an individual's effort to offset feelings of inferiority and establish a sense of adequacy by seeking others' admiration.[7] This is often manifest as grandiosity, intolerance of criticism, and the avoidance of emotional connection, which challenges one's defensive posture. Overly narcissistic individuals may tend to see others as less than full people like themselves, and more as mirrors, potential providers or deniers of psychological affirmation. Their interpersonal world becomes highly personalized, charged, and superficial.

Heinz Kohut and other theorists recognized that some degree of narcissism is a component of everyone's makeup, but in general, relatively little clinical attention is given to status of the self for those who have made the transition to the ordinary subclinical condition of "healthy adult narcissism," because it has been regarded as normal. We recognize that maturation may leaven one's self-centeredness, but we lack a positive alternative conceptualization of the development of self. Consequently, we have not found the tools to address it adequately.

The Psychological Consequences of Ordinary Narcissism

Elements of ordinary narcissism, or "self-belief" as it is called in Buddhism (*sakkaya-ditthi*, in Pali), deserve some description. The unreflective belief in the self naturally gives rise to a natural conviction of our own centrality and importance; we become objects of absolute value.

A number of mischievous consequences follow. Because we identify so strongly with the self, our pleasure or pain is taken *personally*.[8] The world as given takes on a charged quality; that which is pleasurable to me is judged as good, and that which is unpleasant to me is devalued. Our preferences become a yardstick by which all experience is judged, a process that is often so subtle as to remain outside of awareness. We tend to believe our judgments as inevitable and natural responses to events rather than something extra we bring to experience. In a joke my mother used to tell, a young boy asks, "Mom, is that great big piece of cake for Grandma?" "No dear, it's for you." "Aw, what a little hunk."

This selfishness is well described by Venerable Thubten Chodron, a Western nun in the Tibetan Buddhist tradition (n.d.): "It is the attitude that thinks our own happiness is more important than that of everyone else. In its gross form, self-centeredness sees our own ordinary happiness as more important than the happiness of others—it makes us reach for a piece of cake before anyone can get it, cling stubbornly onto our opinions, and get trapped in feelings of guilt." Coupled with less-than-optimal early experience, one is saddled with a lifelong enterprise of maximizing one's own benefit at the expense of others.

It gets worse. The self takes itself as central to all experience, as though it happens to *me*. Once we place the self at the center of psychic life, we seek to render all experience as under our control, to exclude all unpleasant experience and to avoid feeling out of control. This incessant effort is ultimately unsuccessful, and leads to a pervasive sense of unease and restlessness, often in the midst of wonderful or pleasant experience.

To have a sense of separate self is to attribute that same solipsistic quality to all others; in our perception the world becomes populated by separate people and objects, unnaturally isolated in atomistic orbits.[9] A veil of separateness stands between ourselves and others, and within ourselves; we may be left feeling we are standing outside of life.

The fallacy of the self as separate gives rise to insecurity, competition, aggression, jealousy, and defensiveness, all to protect and aggrandize the self. The greatest threat is posed not by eruptions into consciousness of sexuality and aggression, but the fear of one's own insignificance, vulnerability, and mortality (Becker, 1973). Maintenance of one's self-esteem becomes a primary motive in interpersonal and psychic life (Goffman, 1973). This activity is ceaseless, tiresome, and ultimately impossible, because at its root, the Buddhists claim, the one we seek to defend is no more real than a shadow puppet. A Buddhist monk, Achaan Anando, told the following joke (personal communication, February 12, 1987): Question: Why am I unhappy? Answer: Because 99% of everything I think, say, and do is for myself. And there isn't any![10]

NON-SELF, THE THERAPIST, AND THE THERAPEUTIC RELATIONSHIP

Before launching into the benefits that understanding *anatta* brings to the therapeutic relationship, a word of qualification is in order. The assessment of the contribution of the therapist's mindfulness practice is in its infancy. Only a few preliminary empirical studies have been conducted to date, focusing on dimensions that can be measured, such as the therapist's mindfulness and the patient's perception of the therapist's "facilitative qualities" (Wexler, 2006), symptom reduction, and patient evaluation of the treatment (Grepmair et al., 2007). Among Buddhist concepts, *anatta* may remain one of the most elusive to define operationally, as it connotes an *absence* of something; how can absence be measured? In addition, the impact of the direct perception of *anatta* is nearly impossible to disentangle from insight into other key dimensions such as *anicca* (impermanence), or to segregate from other qualities of mind cultivated in meditation. Therefore, the research instrument best suited to this concept may be the idiographic analysis of a single case, that is, one's own experience examined under the microscope of mindful attention.

Ultimately, the self is a concept that we use to organize experience; it has no more substantiality than a thought and, in principle, can be regarded as such, thereby allowing one to escape its familiar gravitational pull. The direct perception of the emptiness of self is hard won through committed meditation practice; no written description or argument can begin to substitute for firsthand experience of *anatta*. As such, it would seem entirely out of reach of the nonmeditating therapist. However, one needn't look to exotic meditation experiences for some clue to the mutability of the self. There is evidence in ordinary experience that points to its "conditional" nature, such as when we are so fully absorbed in focused activity that we forget ourselves even as we are highly alert and engaged (Csikszentmihalyi, 1991), or when the self's activity is absent during deep sleep.

Buddhist literature is replete with accounts of moments of insight that are so adamant that one's perspective of oneself is permanently altered. Among meditators, the experience of the self as insubstantial may take years of practice; indeed, according to Buddhism, full and irreversible liberation from self-view occurs only with the full enlightenment of a buddha. But along the way, those engaged in meditation are rewarded with growing glimpses that are transformative. The unpleasant experience of the self's reaction to—and effort to control—events is readily seen in meditation. When mindfulness and concentration are both strong, we can be fully (though transiently) aware of experience without the accompanying sense of someone to whom it happens.

Such glimpses are rewarded for the way they point to freedom from suffering, both for ourselves and others. In this manner the perception of *anatta* is perfectly compatible with almost any human endeavor (except, perhaps, those that cause harm). The benefit to the therapist of his or her own mindfulness meditation practice, then, is merely one specific instance. But for the clinician's practice of psychotherapy, meditation is invaluable. Even absent such a glimpse into *anatta*, an understanding of the notion can be beneficial to an expanded view of the therapy process. What, then, are these benefits?

As described above, to be a self is to attribute this selfness to others. Such a perspective is natural and common to how we conduct therapy, one self working with another, working to bridge the intersubjective gap. By contrast, to see the nature of self as empty is to reveal it as a process that is utterly inseparable from the rest of life. Though our patients may perceive themselves as isolated, we see this against the larger background in which everything is an inextricable part of everything else. This enables us to see how others' sense of entrapment, often experienced as somehow inevitable, is a product of ignorance of our innate interdependence. As the veil of separateness is lifted, the sense of a world inhabited by separate individuals is replaced by a natural perception of the original condition of connection and intimacy with all we encounter. We don't have to work quite so hard at it; we feel an automatic and uncomplicated affinity with others. This natural affinity is the ideal condition for the creation of the therapeutic relationship, or any other sort of relationship. This extends to our understanding of our patients, whose alienation comes to be seen as a problem of mistaken perception, making it potentially more easily remedied than recovering missed developmental accomplishments.

Just as either the patient's or therapist's mood may set an ambience in the consulting room (of, for example, giddiness, fear, anxiety, warmth, and so on), so does the therapist's grounding in mindfulness influence the tone. Paul Fleischman (1988) described the ambience of *anicca* in the consulting room as both sorrowful (as all change hints of death) and relieving (as all change speaks of possibility). The tone of *anatta* is even less tangible and more transparent, and lies beneath the transient mood of the hour. It may be described as a quality of spaciousness, as though there is ample room for whatever the patient brings, relatively unencumbered by the concern for the therapist's reactivity. Distinguishing between the felt sense of *anicca* and *anatta* is likely a practical impossibility, though Fleischman tries to suggest that patients perceive the spaciousness that characterizes the mind of a long-term meditator. This ambience is suggestive of safety and invitation.

As therapists informed by *anatta*, we learn to hold the conventional view of the self a bit more lightly than is implicit in most psychotherapy. So, even as we help patients to become familiar with themselves, to restore self-esteem, to learn when to confront and when to stand down—that is, doing the familiar work of psychotherapy—we do so while holding the understanding that our patients are far more than their limited self-representations, beneficent or hostile. We become cautious to avoid backing them into a corner, holding them to a view we or they hold of themselves. While we acknowledge authenticity, we become cautious in our use of language to avoid suggesting there is a "true self" at which they can or must arrive. We become allowing of the fact that we are all gloriously inconsistent, and that our need for consistency is obsolete. We don't need to arrive at any final position regarding ourselves, preferring to rest in the natural uncertainty of life. The temptation to conclude that "I'm the kind of person who . . . " should end with " . . . often surprises herself." This flexibility is not just adaptive; it is accurate.

By regarding conventional psychotherapy as a self-building activity (in addition to the less disputable purpose of supporting ego functions), it is easy to conclude that it is inconsistent with the goals of mindfulness as practiced for freedom from delusional self-view. Indeed, it might well be argued that self-restoration and identity consolidation is regressive, reinforcing the very delusion that is at the heart of all suffering, reaffirming our attachment to ourselves as stars of our dramas. However, as Harvey Aronson (2004, p. 84) put it, "To regard therapy as oriented toward *loosening*, and Buddhist insight practice as oriented toward *freeing ourselves from* fixed self-images provides a productive way for understanding the relationship between them." That is, successful treatment may be conducive to movement in the same direction as the path of liberation. Indeed, self-hatred is surely as much an obstacle to liberation as is excessive attachment to positive self-representations. We might hypothesize that it is easier to loosen one's identification with limited self-representations when they are not simultaneously overburdened with self-loathing; even self rejection is a nefarious form of attachment.

This is not to suggest that we use psychotherapy as a vehicle to "enlightenment" or realization of *anatta*, a purpose for which it is ill intended. Some individuals who are drawn to the concept of *anatta* may suffer self-pathology and be in need of skillful psychotherapy. For such individuals, the language of *anatta* may offer comfort as it seems to speak in positive terms to their own sense of diffusion or fragmentation. These maladaptive experiences, however, are not to mistaken for *anatta*, which may require a degree of ego strength as a prerequisite.[11] Mindfulness practice may be disorganizing for these individuals. Even for "healthy narcissists" who do not suffer significant self-pathology, speaking of "not-self" in therapy is likely to leave the patient puzzled, and headed for the door.

To be clear, I do not advocate making *anatta* a clinical principle in the treatment process, yet another theoretical concept against which we judge our patients' experience. I only recommend it to therapists as a *potential*, an alternative perspective from which self-representations are not unduly privileged. Familiarity with the contours of this path is valuable because it can keep the therapist from concluding that a "healthy self" is the last stop. It provides a sense of "next steps" when a patient has gained what there is to gain from psychotherapy, but for whom "ordinary human unhappiness" calls for an existential or spiritual understanding that cannot be adequately provided through symptom-oriented treatment. Efforts to cast such suffering in the personal terms of neurosis may actually be subtly detrimental, as it may suggest treatments that ultimately fail. Not all forms of suffering fall into psychotherapy's range of effectiveness.

As noted above, once we believe the illusion of a separate self, we invest considerable energy aggrandizing and defending the self. This narcissistic activity becomes a source of resistance when it enters into the therapeutic relationship. For instance, we cannot help but feel proud when treatment goes well and we see ourselves reflected as gifted healers in the eyes of our patients. Similarly, we feel shame when treatment appears to go poorly. In short, we are motivated to feel like competent professionals, and our professional self-esteem may seem to be renegotiated anew in every successive session. This may become an obstacle if it begins to interfere with our ability to sit with the fullness of our patient's experience out of our need to be effective. Our wholesome desire to help is trustworthy; our narcissistic *need* to be and be seen as helpful may make us less so. When the self that desires acclaim (from our patients or ourselves) is seen as the empty process that it is, we begin to loosen our grip on the need to protect or defend our professional self-image. We see that anxiety for what it is, and are better equipped to avoid fueling it.

Both Buddhist and Western psychology describe how experience is actively constructed and shaped, rather than passively perceived. Psychoanalytic descriptions of transference highlight one dimension of this coloring of perception in the interpersonal field through their account of how early experience of others is replayed in current relationships, typically outside of conscious awareness. Maladaptive patterns of behavior are repeated because we fail to see how the template of the past distorts the present. Psychotherapy potentially avoids becoming yet another repetition of this pattern by creating an environment in which such transference can be recognized (in some cases, for having been deliberately cultured), and understood. This is only possible when the therapist avoids unwittingly playing the role assigned by his or her patient—that is, countertransference—thereby replicating the very obstacles that beset the patient.

Because transference is usually subtle, its detection requires much of us to avoid becoming enlisted in countertransference due to our own unexamined attachments. Just as an understanding of *anatta* helps reveal our own narcissistic preoccupation, so, too does it provide a degree of protection against becoming lost to transference and countertransference. In the course of becoming adept observers of our own minds and the subtle manipulations of the self, we are learning to *see*. This seeing extends to our perception of others; as we learn to see ourselves more clearly, so does our perception of others seem more vivid for having stilled our own inner chatter through mindfulness practice. Consequently, our clinical formulations arise spontaneously out of the fullness of the moment, rather than as recovered distant memories of psychological theory. By learning to quiet our tendency to grasp for certainty in ideas about ourselves and others, we are more capable of seeing these movements as they arise. When our sly maneuverings are known as nothing more than the reflexive activity of a deluded small self to fortify its imagined privileged position, we can avoid being tripped up, a result much like the desired outcome of a very successful psychoanalysis. Catching ourselves early, we avoid being ensnared by countertransference or enacting our own self-centered dramas with our patients. While remaining utterly present, we learn to get out of the way by not replicating familiar obstacles, thereby creating an open path that patients may or may not choose to travel. They are granted freedom in the therapeutic relationship that they may embrace, as they feel ready.

Seeing the arising of self as a momentary response to conditions, we see how suffering, too, arises in the present moment in response to our clinging. This fine-grained perception of our inner activity enables us to see how each moment is created anew. This perpetual renewal means we are less stuck on a strict deterministic treadmill; freedom becomes imaginable, and this understanding becomes the background of our work with patients. We know what our patients do not yet see, that beyond solving or working through a problem is a more radical sort of relief that doesn't depend on being more or better, ridding oneself of faults, or becoming something different. Hope becomes palpable because we are convinced of the possibility of happiness here and now.

But herein lies a potential problem. This perspective suggests that our suffering arises from a failure to accurately perceive our innate enlightened nature, that we are originally complete. Should the therapist rest unreflectively on such a view, he or she may hold the patient's suffering too lightly as also being ultimately insubstantial and happening to "no one," thereby not taking it seriously enough.[12] The patient may experience the therapist's stance as an empathic departure. Good clinical judgment and genuine empathy are as essential here as in any successful therapy.

CONCLUSION

The juxtaposition of Buddhist and Western psychological concepts in theory and in clinical practice invites a number of intriguing questions. We might be tempted to wonder whether the Buddhist or the Western psychological understanding of self might ultimately be revealed as more "accurate," or alternatively, conclude that they remain incompatible and irreconcilable for deriving their meaning entirely from their unique cultural and philosophical contexts. But the increasing appropriation of mindfulness as an adjunct to psychotherapy has created a new context. When an individual engages in both psychotherapy and Buddhist meditation, must we invoke two models of understanding to account for changes to one person? Might these practices address different "levels" of psychic organization, suggesting that the self of Western psychology and the self challenged by *anatta* are evidence of multiple—potentially nonintersecting—selves? Is it accurate to posit *anatta* as an extension of self development described in Western psychology? In time, might we forge a model of personality that embraces an adaptive role for *anatta*? Can this be accomplished without reductionism? How would such a conception influence psychotherapy's techniques? One crucible for this experiment is the shared experience of therapist and patient in the consulting room; another is the private inner life of the meditating patient. Both are now generating new material for active consideration.

These questions need not await resolution for the clinician to benefit from an understanding of *anatta*, nor do we hurriedly need to create a Buddhist psychotherapy. *Anatta*, understood by the therapist, remains effectively invisible and should not be construed as a new set of techniques or theory. Indeed, it suggests that we hold *any* new perspective—including a Buddhist perspective—more lightly and cautiously, as we understand the dangers of taking any fixed position that we must then work to protect, or work to relinquish.

NOTES

1. As this volume attests, *anatta* is only one facet of mindfulness that can be of great value to the therapist. To isolate *anatta* for special consideration without reference to the larger context of Buddhist psychology is a bit suspect. It is hoped the reader understands this rather unnaturally narrow focus as a response to the relative neglect of *anatta* in recent efforts to introduce mindfulness to the clinical setting.
2. Ethological research with primates, dolphins, and elephants is beginning to challenge this vestige of human conceit.
3. As philosopher Ernst Cassirer put it (1955, p. 156), "The crucial achievement of every symbolic form lies precisely in the fact that it does not have the limit between I and reality as pre-existent and established for all time but must itself create this line—and that each fundamental form creates it in a different way."
4. Prominent proponents of this view include social interactionists such as George Herbert Mead, Emile Durkheim, and Erving Goffman.
5. Within Buddhist philosophy, the ontological status of the self has been hotly debated for many centuries, without consensus. It is outside the scope of this article to explore some of the finer points of this debate. Interested readers might begin with an excellent discussion by Harvey Aronson (2004), who is

both a psychotherapist and Buddhist scholar, and Barry Magid (2002), who is
both a Zen teacher and psychoanalyst.

6. Buddhist psychological literature deconstructs the experience of self in a number of ways. For example, in some literature it is described as an assemblage of
parts and processes (*khandas* in Pali), no one of which is the sole essential ingredient. Elsewhere it is analyzed as a recursive feedback loop describing the
conditions that give rise to the experience (*paticca-samuppada* in Pali). An excellent description of this can be found in Olendzki (2005).

7. For some, narcissism may not be a defense against feelings of inferiority; they
may simply love themselves more than most. See Wink (1991) for a discussion
of "overt" and "covert" narcissism.

8. In the Buddhist formulation, the reaction to pleasant or unpleasant stimuli is
actually antecedent to the momentary arising of the sense of self, generated by
the nearly instinctive reaction of grasping or pushing away, in consonance with
the pleasure principle.

9. In the words of Sri Nisargadatta Maharaj (1973, p. 37), "When you believe
yourself to be a person, you see persons everywhere."

10. Of course, having a self is no small accomplishment, and its existence can be attributed to the adaptive purposes it serves. Indeed, the achievement of various
culturally consonant qualities of self, well represented in clinical theory, are essential ingredients of adjustment; for many, learning assertiveness, cohesive-
ness, self-regard, and good boundaries are essential for well-being. This admit-
tedly one-sided account is intended to highlight the less acknowledged ways
even a "healthy self" is a source of suffering.

11. See Engler (2003) for an excellent discussion of this topic.

12. This is a facet of what is sometimes described as "attachment to emptiness" in
Mahayana Buddhism.

REFERENCES

Aronson, H. (2004). *Buddhist practice on Western ground*. Boston: Shambhala.

Becker, E. (1973). *The denial of death*. New York: Free Press.

Beneviste, E. (1971). *Problems in general linguistics* (Miami Linguistic Series, no. 8). Coral
Gables, FL: University of Miami Press.

Bohm, D. (1973). Human nature as the product of our mental models. In J. Benthall (Ed.),
The limits of human nature (pp. 92–114). New York: Dutton.

Cassirer, E. (1955). *The philosophy of symbolic forms: Vol. 2. Mythical thought*. New Haven,
CT: Yale University Press.

Chodron, Thubten, Ven. (n.d.). Ego: A Tibetan perspective. Retrieved February 11, 2007,
from *purifymind.com/TibetanPerspective.htm*.

Crapanzano, V. (1979). The self, the third, and desire. In B. Lee (Ed.), *Psychosocial theories
of the self* (pp. 179–206). New York: Plenum Press.

Csikszentmihalyi, M. (1991). *Flow*. New York: HarperCollins.

Engler, J. (2003). Being somebody and being nobody: A reexamination of the understanding of self in psychoanalysis and Buddhism. In J. Safran (Ed.), *Psychoanalysis and Buddhism* (pp. 35–79). Boston: Wisdom.

Fleischman, P. (1988). Awareness of *anicca* and the practice of psychotherapy. *Journal of Contemplative Psychotherapy, 5,* 43–52.

Gallimore, R. (1981). Affiliation, social context, industriousness, and achievement. In R. H. Munroe, R. L. Munroe, & B. B. Whiting (Eds.), *Handbook of cross-cultural human development* (pp. 689–715). New York: Garland.

Goffman, E. (1973). *The presentation of self in everyday life.* Woodstock, NY: Overlook Press.

Grepmair, L., Mitterlehner, F., Loew, T., Bachler, E., Rother, W., & Nickel, M. (2007). Promoting mindfulness in psychotherapists in training influences the treatment results of their patients: A randomized, double-blind, controlled study. *Psychotherapy and Psychosomatics, 76*(6), 332–338.

Hallowell, I. (1955). *Culture and experience.* Philadelphia: University of Pennsylvania Press.

Kernberg, O. (1975). *Borderline conditions and pathological narcissism.* New York: Jason Aronson.

Kohut, H. (1977). *The restoration of the self.* New York: International Universities Press.

Lasch, C. (1979). *The culture of narcissism: American life in an age of diminishing expectations.* New York: Norton.

Lee, D. (1959). *Freedom and culture.* Englewood Cliffs, NJ: Prentice-Hall.

Levy-Bruhl, L. (1928). *The "soul" of the primitive.* New York: Macmillan.

Magid, B. (2002). *Ordinary mind: Exploring the common ground of Zen and psychotherapy.* Boston: Wisdom.

Maharaj, S. N. (1973). *I am that* (Trans. M. Frydman). Bombay: Chetana.

Mead, G. H. (1932). *Mind, self, and society.* Chicago: University of Chicago Press.

Olendzki, A. (2005). The roots of mindfulness. In C. Germer, R. Siegel, & P. Fulton (Eds.), *Mindfulness and psychotherapy* (pp. 241–261). New York: Guilford Press.

Schweder, R., & Bourne, E. J. (1982). Does the concept of the person vary cross-culturally? In A. Marcella & G. M. White (Eds.), *Cultural conceptions of mental health and therapy.* Dordrecht, the Netherlands: D. Reidel.

Tseng, W. (1978). Traditional and modern psychiatric care in Taiwan. In A. Kleinman, P. Kunstadter, E. Alexander, & J. Gale (Eds.), *Culture and healing in Asian societies: Anthropological, psychiatric, and public health studies* (pp. 311–328). Cambridge, MA: Schenkman.

Wexler, J. (2006). *Therapist mindfulness and the therapeutic alliance.* Unpublished manuscript, Massachusetts School of Professional Psychology, Boston, MA.

Wink, P. (1991). Two faces of narcissism. *Journal of Personality and Social Psychology, 61,* 590–597.

5 Mindfulness and Empathy

A Hermeneutic Circle

RUSSELL A. WALSH

In the beginner's mind there are many possibilities,
but in the expert's there are few.
—SHUNRYU SUZUKI (1970, p. 21)

This chapter discusses the problematic nature of empathy, the promise of mindfulness as remedy, and the implications of both for the training of therapists. To explore the possibility, and potential impossibility, of empathy, I draw upon the work of humanistic and phenomenological scholars with the goal of discerning the hermeneutic or interpretive character of empathy. I then sketch out, both theoretically and practically, the benefits of mindfulness for disclosing the therapist's presence in any attempt at understanding. From there I describe how reflective listening exercises, informed by hermeneutics and mindfulness practices, can provide a foundation for the training and ongoing professional development of therapists.

Virtually every approach to psychotherapy or counseling acknowledges the importance of empathy. As one of the common factors of psychotherapy and counseling (Lambert & Bergin, 1994; see also Lambert & Simon, Chapter 2, this volume), empathy is recognized either as a setting operation from which effective interventions may follow or as the central ingredient that promotes reflection and change. Accordingly, a key component of most psychotherapy or counseling training programs is a process for facilitating the development of therapist empathy.

But if empathy is so important, then how does one teach, and learn, it? It seems that most efforts to promote the development of empathy are based on either one or both of two assumptions. The first is that empathy is an innate ability that can be called upon and refined through conscious effort. The second is that empathy is a skill that can be learned, and improved upon, through repeated practice. It is probably a combination of these beliefs that underpins reflective listening exercises, wherein therapists in training are instructed to repeat verbatim key words and phrases from their clients' discourse, allowing the clients to either affirm or correct the therapists' reflections.

As a clinical approach, reflective listening is supposed to keep the therapist focused on the client's experience and to communicate to the client the therapist's effort to understand. It invites clients to hear and consider their own characterizations of experience, and thereby reflectively listen to themselves. As a pedagogical strategy, reflective listening exercises are designed to foster the therapist in training's attunement to others, with the presumed result of increasing the capacity for empathy. However, the increased self-awareness that reflective listening offers clients may be equally important for therapists in training (as well as for experienced therapists), particularly with regard to the development of empathy. If empathy is a relational endeavor, then it depends on the therapist's, as well as the client's, openness to discovery. Hence reflective listening exercises should entail both listening to and reflecting back to the client as well as listening to and reflecting on one's position as a therapist. This latter function of reflective listening, and the crucial role of self-awareness in any empathic endeavor, will be explored both theoretically and practically in this chapter.

REFLECTIVE LISTENING AND EMPATHY: THE PROBLEM WITH GETTING IT RIGHT

What is perhaps most remarkable about reflective listening exercises is the speed with which therapists in training are moved through and beyond these practices. In my own experience, six to eight 10-minute sessions with a fellow student were presumed to be sufficient to build a foundation for empathy. As a clinical supervisor and course instructor, I recognize the challenge of too many issues in too little time when trying to provide a solid foundation for beginning therapists. Still, I have to admit that few therapists in training have the slightest glimpse of what empathy might be at the conclusion of introductory exercises. To be honest, after 20 years of clinical practice, empathy still remains for me a beguiling and bewildering process.

In my efforts to teach both myself and my students what empathic presence might look and feel like, here is one of the problems I've encountered: It seems that those who claim to "get it right" are often furthest from the mark. In other words, it is with those students for whom understanding seems straightforward that I am most concerned. And the same is true of experienced therapists. As psychotherapy client and professional colleague, I have often encountered therapists who presume to be empathic but in fact seem to understand very little. Moreover, in my own work as a therapist I have been humbled by the times when my empathic grasp of a client's experience has been torn apart by disconfirming evidence. The humbling aspect of this is not that it occurs, but that it highlights the unknown frequency with which my many empathic moments weren't torn apart but should have been. As LeShan (1996, p. 54), citing his mentor Abraham Meyerson, warns:

> As soon as you have decided, on the basis of long experience and sound theory, that all patients who have "A" also have "B," within three days some character will come into your office with "A" but without "B." The big question is not whether or not this will happen—it will—but whether or not you will notice it!

This paradox—that more experience as a therapist may pose an obstacle to empathy—was echoed in research on the development of psychotherapists' values over the course of psychotherapy training (Walsh, Perrucci, & Severns, 1999). Comparing beginning therapists in training to those at more advanced levels, we found that participants' valuing of empathy seemed to fall with increased training. Whether this reflected participants devaluing empathy or merely taking it for granted, it suggests that empathy is not something that necessarily improves over time.

Another example regarding the complicated nature of empathy can be found in Fessler's (1983) research on the psychotherapy process. In one of the first published studies comparing therapist and client accounts of their psychotherapy sessions, Fessler found that a moment of understanding from the therapist's point of view was experienced quite differently by the client. Specifically, what the therapist described as empathic attunement and interpretation that broke through the client's resistance was characterized in these words by the client: "I thought he didn't know what the hell he was talking about" (p. 43).

Empathy, in other words, is a problematic concept. While recognized as a key feature of effective psychotherapy, it is neither a capacity that unfolds naturally nor a skill that develops with a clear and positive trajectory. It may in fact degrade or slip away over time. And it may be that our subjective sense of getting it, that is, of genuinely being empathic, correlates little or not at all with the client's experience of being understood. So where do we go from here?

BACK TO CARL ROGERS

Perhaps we should return to Carl Rogers, who coined the phrase *accurate empathy* in his formulation of humanistic psychotherapy. It is notable that Rogers's term includes the qualifier *accurate*, presumably allowing for the converse: inaccurate empathy. In his characterization of accurate empathy, Rogers (1992) said:

> To sense the client's private world as if it were your own, but without ever losing the "as if" quality—this is empathy, and this seems essential to therapy. To sense the client's anger, fear, or confusion as if it were your own, yet without your own anger, fear, or confusion getting bound up in it, is the condition we are endeavoring to describe. (p. 832)

Hence one defining feature of accurate empathy is sensing the client's private experience as if it were your own, without forgetting what Rogers calls the "as if" quality of this effort. Although Rogers does not elaborate on this, I would suggest that this "as if" quality entails recognizing that one's sense of the client's experience is always a projection based at least in part on one's own experience. However, this suggestion is complicated by Rogers's second defining feature of accurate empathy. Here a precise distinction is made between the client's experience and the therapist's experience, with the intermingling of the two seen as problematic.

In light of Roger's characterizations of accurate empathy, we can suppose that inaccurate empathy would occur when the therapist presumes to understand or imposes his or her understanding on the client. Accordingly, we could say that the accuracy of empathy depends on the degree to which it is freed from the presuppositions of the therapist. This characterization, however, would place us directly on a collision course with phenomenology—an approach with which Rogers saw his work deeply allied. Hence clarifying and exploring a solution to inaccurate empathy will require a detour through the fields of phenomenology and hermeneutics.

PHENOMENOLOGY AND HERMENEUTICS

Phenomenological psychology (Giorgi, Fischer, & Von Eckartsberg, 1971; Giorgi, Fischer, & Murray, 1975; Giorgi, Knowles, & Smith, 1979; Giorgi, Barton, & Maes, 1983) is concerned with grounding the scientific understandings of human beings in the lived experience of human beings. Heralding Edmund Husserl's (1900) dictum, "to the things themselves," phenomenological psychologists have favored first-person accounts of experiences over abstract theoretical or quantitative representations of those experiences. Through qualitative methods of interpretation, phenomenologists strive to identify core features or characteristics of human existence so that an appropriately human science, based on lived experience, can inform psychological knowledge.

Phenomenology underscores the problematic notion of objectivity and the inadequacy of a detached, reductionistic posture for making sense of human experience. Privileging understanding over prediction and control, phenomenologists embrace the complex interplay of consciousness, context, and embodiment through which human experience occurs.

Rogers's desire to remain faithful to the lived experience of his clients is what led him to use the term *phenomenological* to describe his client-centered approach. However, Rogers did not really concern himself with the interpretive aspect of phenomenology—an aspect that has grown in importance over the past several decades, to the point where the term *hermeneutic phenomenology*, or simply *hermeneutics*, has become a dominant trope. Rather, in positioning humanistic psychology in contradistinction to psychoanalysis, Rogers saw client-centered therapy—with its foundation of accurate empathy, unconditional positive regard, and genuineness—as an alternative to interpretation. Hence for Rogers these features of the humanistic attitude were a means for understanding the experiences of clients without imposing the therapist's interpretive bias on that understanding.

Over the past several decades, the ideal of attaining understanding free from bias has been whittled away by many phenomenologists, most significantly Martin Heidegger and Hans-Gorge Gadamer. These two thinkers highlighted the engaged, contextual, and bias-laden nature of any understanding—even, perhaps especially, those attempts to understand by remaining free from bias.

Heidegger (1927/1962) pointed out that the inherently contextual nature of experience is such that our apprehension and understanding of any phenomenon (person, event, experience, etc.) is defined by the clearing within which it emerges for us. This clearing is a background, both in the sense that our understanding of a figure is contingent on its surroundings, and in the sense that the surroundings, while foundational, are less clear or even invisible to the perceiver. Hence presuppositions are defining features of, rather than obstacles to, our empathic understanding.

Gadamer (1975) further underscored how biases or presuppositions are the means through which understanding is made possible. When we seek to make sense of anything (or anyone), we do so by virtue of our own frame of reference. While this frame of reference can be expanded and modified over time (think of Piaget's notion of accommodation), it is by its nature inseparable from understanding. Hence any effort to set aside or reject one's bias is as likely to ignore or repress the impact of that bias. As an alternative, human science advocates recommend the exploration and clarification of biases that are manifested in our efforts to understand. This ongoing dialectic between seeking to understand and recognizing one's biases has been characterized as the hermeneutic circle.

EMPATHY AND THE HERMENEUTIC CIRCLE

The term *hermeneutic circle* highlights the interaction or clash between empathic projection—the imposition of assumptions in an attempt to understand—and the inadequacy of that projection to the lived experience of those persons whom we are trying to understand. With each attempt at empathy, listeners are (or should be, at least) made aware of how little they do in fact understand. As a result, each pass through the circle leads to greater uncertainty about the other along with increased sensitivity to the biases that are projected. This in turn leads to further scrutiny of those presuppositions, an increasingly complex picture of the other, and subsequent attempts to project further understanding.

The compass for navigating through the hermeneutic circle is composed of reflection, skepticism, and humility. Phrased differently, we could say that *in the moments when therapists believe with certainty that they understand something, they may in fact have lost their way.* The circular nature of interpretation is such that understanding is never achieved in any absolute sense. Rather, it is the ultimate impossibility of understanding that keeps the reflective process going. Hence, while therapists may gain a deeper appreciation for the complexity of their clients' experience, that appreciation should be accompanied by an equally growing sense of humility and awe in the face of that experience.

So understanding, to the degree it is achieved at all, is a highly tentative process that consists more of not knowing than of knowing. But the humbling aspect of this process may run counter to the typical trajectory of therapists and therapists in training. Whether or not repeated practice (via reflective listening exercises or accumulated therapeutic experience) improves one's attunement to others, it is likely that it fosters in the listener an increased sense of competence. This sense of competence—a particularly welcome achievement for therapists in training—may jeopardize empathy in several ways. First, it may lead to the presumption of understanding and a lack of humility and reflection. Second, an increased sense of competence may shape the conversation between therapist and client in undesirable ways. Here it is worth noting that Gadamer (1975) distinguished between what he called speculative language, or language that opens up or reveals possibilities, and statements, which distort experience through precision. According to Gadamer, the latter occur when the encounter between listener and speaker becomes interrogative—for which a central feature is the authority and confidence of the interviewer (Walsh, 2004).

The hermeneutic circle can counter the dark side of competence by returning the therapist again and again to the surprising and contradictory aspects of each client's lived experience. In a sense, this is a return to each present moment, which is necessarily fuller and more complex than any formulation of experience. This repeated return to the present moment invites both the therapist and the client to remain open to surprise and spontaneity, and thereby experience themselves (individually and collectively) in novel ways.

Within the human sciences, there is debate about where the hermeneutic circle ultimately leads. Does the back and forth movement through one's biases and one's attempts to understand ever end? While for most the answer to this ultimate question would be no, there are those who characterize the hermeneutic circle as a spiral, increasing in depth with each revolution. Hence despite the potential for false confidence over time, there may also be growth of self-awareness and appreciation for the complexity of understanding. With regard to empathy, if there is anything like wisdom, it is likely to be a capacity to embrace and stand humbled before the awesome and ultimately impossible task of truly understanding another person.

Although humanistic psychology was developed as a remedy to the objectifying propensities of other psychotherapeutic approaches, without sufficient humility and skepticism it can produce what Richer has called the humanistic "secret police" (1992). Confident in our genuineness and empathic abilities, we run the risk of imposing our values and assumptions in a way that is hidden from our (and perhaps our clients') awareness. Hence the hermeneutic circle serves as a reminder of our indelible presence in any empathic move as well as a process for examining and owning that presence.

Viewed hermeneutically, the practice of empathy should focus as much on recognizing the therapist's biases as on accessing the client's experience. The challenge of course is finding a stance, or attitude, by which to navigate that hermeneutic circle. It is this task of balancing nonjudgmental acceptance of one's biases with openness to the present moment for which mindfulness seems ideally suited.

MINDFULNESS AND THE HERMENEUTIC CIRCLE

Within the fields of phenomenology and hermeneutics, there has been little discussion of obstacles to the reflection and humility that are called for methodologically. As Heidegger pointed out, when we are engaged in activity—including the activity of listening—we are by nature unreflective. Moreover, the stance we undertake when reflecting on our experience requires a certain degree of detachment from that engaged activity. While Heidegger and others have highlighted this distinction, few human science scholars have proposed precisely how one might hover over, or vacillate between, these differing modes of engagement. One exception in this regard is Adams (1995), who called attention to the similarities between the phenomenological posture known as bracketing, the psychoanalytic concept of evenly hovering attention and the meditative stance of "revelatory openness wedded with the clarity of unknowing," (p. 465). In this thoughtful paper, Adams points to the crucial role of nonjudgmental acceptance and tolerance of not knowing within each of these traditions.

Whereas phenomenology employs the concept of the thing in itself, Buddhists use the term *tathata*, meaning reality in itself or suchness. The method for attaining suchness is mindfulness. Generally speaking, we could say that mindfulness practices entail returning again and again to a point of focus while recognizing and accepting the flow of thoughts and emotions that clutter each present moment. The first, and some might say the only, step in these practices is nonjudgmental acceptance of the clutter along with continued effort to embrace the present moment. This dance is necessarily circular, in that vacillating between self-reflection and presence is an ongoing and never-ending process. The goal of this process is the process itself, with each pass through the circle inviting a deeper appreciation for the complexity and beauty of every moment.

Although the word *mindfulness* is seldom used in discussions of phenomenology and the hermeneutic circle, it seems clear that the interpretive process is hopeless and potentially dangerous without the grounding stance of mindfulness. It is only by recognizing and accepting the inevitable imposition of ourselves (including our assumptions, expectations, fears, and ambitions) in any effort to understand that we have a chance of connecting with another person, and of being challenged, confused, and surprised by the complex individual who stands before us. And without confusion and surprise any empathic move may be little more than assimilating the whole of the client before us into a set of assumptions with which we are most familiar and comfortable.

If mindfulness does not facilitate understanding in any definitive sense, it provides an entry point for the dance of self-reflection and presence. Moreover, as this dance is one easily abandoned in favor of familiar steps, mindfulness provides a stance to which one can return again and again in order to begin anew. This process of nonjudgmental acceptance, reflection, and repeated return to the present moment is an ideal medium in which empathy can be nurtured and grown.

MINDFULNESS AND EMPATHY

I began this chapter with the question "How does one teach, and learn, empathy?" Now that we've explored both the complicated nature of empathy and the promise of mindfulness for the hermeneutic circle, I will venture an answer. A mindful and hermeneutical approach to teaching and learning about empathy might begin with reexamining assumptions about the nature of empathy. As discussed at the start of this chapter, one foundational assumption is that empathy is an innate ability that can be called upon through conscious effort. A mindful, hermeneutical approach would qualify this claim by specifying both the nature of empathy and the type of conscious effort that is called for. If empathy is an innate capacity, like most human capacities it has both positive and negative potentials. Relying unquestioningly on its accuracy neglects the oppressive potential of understanding. Hence the conscious effort required to develop or refine the capacity for empathy must be grounded by self-reflection and humility.

The second foundational assumption—that empathy is a skill one can learn and improve upon through practice—must also be modified in a mindfulness-based hermeneutical approach. Like enlightenment, empathy can be seen as an ideal that is impossible in an absolute sense. Nonetheless, it remains an ideal of which we can attain glimpses in moments of presence and self-awareness. Hence practices that facilitate self-awareness and presence provide both a path toward the ideal and a method for experiencing the wondrous clutter that surrounds that path. If improvement occurs at all in this mindful process, it is more in the acceptance of the clutter than in its ultimate transcendence.

Within this revised approach to empathy, teaching entails deconstructing, or shaking up, the presumption of understanding, and recognizing the biases through which understanding is undertaken. Both the process and desired outcome of this approach are comprised of insecurity, humility, and awe along with thoughtfulness, openness, and compassion. It provides a point of focus to which the therapist-in-training can return again and again, and a means for attending to the clutter that surrounds that point of focus. In other words, the teaching of empathy might better be characterized as inviting and facilitating mindfulness.

Let's consider a common mindfulness exercise. The student is instructed to attend to his or her breath, perhaps counting the breath with each exhale. At one level this instruction is impossible to follow, as the student's attention will soon veer from the breath to any number of distracting thoughts and feelings. The teacher—once the student is brave enough to acknowledge his or her failing—will instruct the student to allow and notice the distracting thoughts and feelings while returning to the breath again and again. If the student is anything like me, he or she will return to the task of meditation determined to get it right, and will be frustrated by the experience of recognizing (and judging) again and again the many undesirable thoughts and feelings that pose obstacles to the task of following the breath. The student, in other words, will mistake the goals of meditation as purity and precision rather than as self-knowledge and acceptance. And only by facing repeatedly the assumptions and judgments that shape his or her identity will the student become better able to see, hear, and be present to the complexities of the surrounding world.

Now let's consider reflective listening exercises, and the ways in which they can be taken up as meditative practices. When provided with instruction in these exercises, students are typically urged to faithfully repeat the words and phrases of their clients (or colleagues in the client role). These instructions identify as a point of focus the discourse and experience of the client. In response to this instruction, students will either fail miserably or succeed at all costs. In other words, students will either become aware of their presence in every attempt at understanding or they will become attached to the precision of their reflective listening and, as a result, remain blinded to the complexity—in a precise sense, impossibility—of accurate empathy.

Mindful reflective listening involves listening reflectively to our biases as they are manifested in our efforts to understand. Like clouds moving across the sky, these presuppositions can be noticed, accepted without judgment, and allowed to pass again from view (back to the background) for an expanded perspective on ourselves and on the client who sits before us. Hence we return again and again to the present moment, with an increasingly clearer sense of who we are as listeners. And as a result we gain a deeper appreciation of both how and to whom we are listening.

As with many meditative practices, the student must struggle with his or her desire for perfection and consequent difficulty in acknowledging shortcomings. Despite a teacher's encouragement to let go, the student may want to get it right and win the teacher's approval. Hence the structure of many practices holds the dual functions of facilitating present awareness and letting go along with opening the student to his or her self-criticism and desire for perfection.

In practice, what might all this mean for the training of therapists? In my work as an instructor of therapists in training, I begin by reading and discussing some writings of Carl Rogers, along with other readings addressing the complexity and in some senses impossibility of psychotherapy. I wonder aloud with my students about the term *accurate empathy* and consider how the term may make understanding an ideal that is ultimately unattainable. We discuss how humbling it can be when faced with this impossible goal, and underscore the value of that humility. In this regard we explore the subjective sense of "I understand" as a valuable indicator of *inaccurate* empathy. Calling to mind personal instances when each of us has experienced in a hurtful way someone's insistence that they understand us, we discuss the arrogance of presumptive understanding as well as the potential for each of us to find comfort in that arrogance. As a remedy for the deluded path of arrogant empathy, we agree to undertake a series of exercises to facilitate humility and self-awareness. From this position, we begin reflective listening exercises.

We undertake reflective listening exercises with the expectation that all exercises will be audiotaped or videotaped, and that students will transcribe the full interplay of conversation between themselves and their clients (or persons in the client role). We discuss Heidegger's argument that we can reflect on our mode of engagement only when something breaks down, or when a problem is encountered. Hence the task presented to the students entails scrutinizing their transcribed sessions and identifying either points where they veered beyond reflective listening (often to advice giving or consoling) or where they "got it right" (hence wrong) and presumed to understand. These instances are offered for class discussion, with the overarching question "what does this encounter reveal about me as a listener?"

Repeating the exercise with many colleagues, and experiencing the impact of others' attempts to understand (when in the role of client), students are encouraged to refine the overarching question by considering how they are consistent in their efforts to understand as well as how their efforts change with each unique client. Over the course of these exercises students may improve at reflective listening. But that, of course, is beside the point. Just as the outcome of successive breath awareness may in fact be greater focus on the breath, it is the process of "polishing the mirror" that allows for greater openness and moment-by-moment awareness.

I've found that audiotaping, videotaping, and particularly transcribing offer unique opportunities for facilitating mindfulness. As everyone who has listened to themselves or observed themselves on tape knows, there is nothing more decentering and humbling than this experience. It challenges our sense of who we are and invites us to see aspects of ourselves with which we are unfamiliar or uncomfortable. Transcribing exacerbates this process, both by requiring careful scrutiny of ourselves and attending in particularly to the gap between what we say and what we think we say. A further benefit of transcribing is an increased to sensitivity to the power of language, and the unique ways in which clients and therapists enter and negotiate a conversation.

The format of these exercises is akin to the decentering structure of the student–teacher relationship in Zen Buddhism. Within a context that calls for students to seek improvement and approval, they are instructed to follow a directive (listen reflectively!), yet accept and share proudly their failures in this regard. Moreover, when they do seem to get it right, they are reminded that they are probably getting it wrong, and must therefore explore how their apparent success could reflect an underlying empathic failure. In this way the seemingly straightforward process of reflective listening is made a practice in humility, self-reflection, and surrender to the complexity of each client–therapist encounter.

THE CONTEXT OF MINDFUL EMPATHY

Having considered the complexity of accurate empathy, we should return—as good phenomenologists—to its broader context. For Rogers (1961) accurate empathy could only be manifested in a *relationship* between therapist and client—a relationship further characterized by the therapist's genuineness and unconditional positive regard for the client. In another chapter, at another time, we could similarly explore the ideal or impossible nature of these other factors. But for now it must suffice for us to note that, like empathy, these ideals provide the path for a never-ending journey. And this journey, like all journeys, is not traveled alone.

The therapeutic relationship is a particular kind of relationship, one that exists explicitly for the client. The ethical imperatives that accompany this relationship for the other include a kind of selflessness and surrender summarized eloquently by R. D. Walsh (2005, p. 34):

> You sit across from me in the small room. I do not know definitively who you are. I do not know what I am doing exactly or what will happen next, but I am open to it. Together we are groping in the dark for some illumination from the process itself, from what is happening here and now for us that, if we allow it, if we are patient, will show us the next thing to be done; discerning together because we must, because it is better than groping alone (which is impossible anyway), because this is what we find ourselves doing as if compelled, as if moved by something outside us, passionately, subjectively, with little comfort from any theoretical understanding and knowledge which always arrives too late upon the scene to heal anything—yet with overflowing desire for the health and wholeness and well-being of the other.

This surrender is one of openness, humility, and acceptance of both the client's and the therapist's imperfect human presence. And the selflessness accompanying it is not a naive quest to set aside one's self for the sake of pristine understanding. Instead, it is a careful acceptance of the responsibility and complexity of trying to understand, along with a willingness to return again and again to one's presuppositions and the disconfirming presence of the client. This process, in other words, can also be characterized as the hermeneutic circle of mindfulness and empathy.

CONCLUSION

While empathy is widely acknowledged to be a crucial component of effective psychotherapy, the problematic nature of understanding makes both the training and practice of empathy complex endeavors. This chapter describes the problem of presumptive understanding and its implications for the ideal of empathy. Put briefly, when we as therapists believe we've achieved empathy we are most likely to be imposing our fantasy of understanding on our clients. A potential corrective to this problem is provided by developments in the theoretical conceptualization of understanding in the fields of phenomenology and hermeneutics, particularly with regard to the notion of bias and its role in understanding.

The hermeneutic circle, or dialectical interplay between the presuppositions that frame understanding and the contradictory presence one seeks to understand, shows empathy to be a gradual, complicated, ever-deepening, and ultimately unending process. Using mindfulness as a means for navigating the uncertain journey of empathy can train psychotherapists to cultivate a stance of doubly reflective listening, or attending to both their clients and their own complicated presence as listeners. Reflective listening exercises, often a formative component of psychotherapist training programs, can be reformulated in light of mindfulness and the hermeneutic circle, with inaccurate empathy presented as an important point of focus. Finally, it is important to remember that the possibility of empathy resides in the broader context of a relationship between client and therapist, and that this relationship, like any relationship, is a complicated and co-constituted adventure.

REFERENCES

Adams, W. (1995). Revelatory openness wedded with the clarity of unknowing: Psychoanalytic evenly suspended attention, the phenomenological attitude, and meditative awareness. *Psychoanalysis and Contemporary Thought, 18*(4), 463–494.

Fessler, R. (1983). Phenomenology and "the talking cure": Research on psychotherapy. In

A. Giorgi, A. Barton, & C. Maes (Eds.), *Duquesne studies in phenomenological psychology* (Vol. 4, pp. 33–46). Pittsburgh: Duquesne University Press.

Gadamer, H. (1975). *Truth and method.* New York: Continuum.

Giorgi, A., Barton, A., & Maes, C. (1983). *Duquesne studies in phenomenological psychology* (Vol. 4). Pittsburgh: Duquesne University Press.

Giorgi, A., Fischer, C., & Murray, E. (1975). *Duquesne studies in phenomenological psychology* (Vol. 2). Pittsburgh: Duquesne University Press.

Giorgi, A., Fischer, W. F., & Von Eckartsberg, R. (1971). *Duquesne studies in phenomenological psychology* (Vol. 1). Pittsburgh: Duquesne University Press.

Giorgi, A., Knowles, R., & Smith, D. (1979). *Duquesne studies in phenomenological psychology* (Vol. 3). Pittsburgh: Duquesne University Press.

Heidegger, M. (1962). *Being and time.* New York: Harper & Row. (Original work published 1927)

Husserl, E. (1900). *Logical investigations.* New York: Humanities Press.

Lambert, M. J., & Bergin, A. (1994). The effectiveness of psychotherapy. In S. Garfield & A. Bergin (Eds.), *Handbook of psychotherapy and behavior change* (pp. 143–189). New York: Wiley.

LeShan, L. (1996). *Beyond technique: Psychotherapy for the 21st century.* Northvale, NJ: Jason Aronson.

Richer, P. (1992). An introduction to deconstructionist psychology. In S. Kvale (Ed.), *Psychology and postmodernism.* London: Sage.

Rogers, C. (1961). *On becoming a person.* Boston: Houghton Mifflin.

Rogers, C. (1992). The necessary and sufficient conditions of therapeutic personality change. *Journal of Consulting and Clinical Psychology, 60*(6), 827–832.

Suzuki, S. (1970). *Zen mind, beginner's mind: Informal talks on Zen meditation and practice.* New York: Weatherhill.

Walsh, R. A. (2004). The methodological implications of Gadamer's distinction between statements and speculative language. *Humanistic Psychologist, 32*(2), 105–119.

Walsh, R. A., Perrucci, A., & Severns, J. (1999). What's in a good moment: Hermeneutic study of psychotherapy values across levels of psychotherapy training. *Psychotherapy Research, 9*(3), 304–326.

Walsh, R. D. (2005). Beyond therapy: Levinas and ethical therapeutics. *European Journal of Psychotherapy, Counselling and Health, 7*(1–2), 29–35.

III THERAPEUTIC PRESENCE IN DIFFERENT TYPES OF TREATMENT

Coming from such different approaches, one might think that the authors of these chapters would have quite different understandings of the therapeutic relationship. And indeed, there are differences of nuance among them. But the similarities are far more striking. All the authors in this section, whether coming from a behavioral foundation, like Kelly Wilson and Emily Sandoz, and G. Alan Marlatt, Sarah Bowen, Neha Chawla, and Katie Witkiewitz, or from a psychoanalytic base, like Jeremy Safran and Romy Reading, or from a family therapy perspective like Mishka Lysack, emphasize deep human connectedness, devoid of the detached role of the expert. In all there is a sense that the therapeutic relationship is co-created, that it is first of all and above all else, a decent human relationship.

Wilson and Sandoz discuss the therapeutic relationship in the context of acceptance and commitment therapy (ACT), stressing the importance of seeing the client as more like a sunset than a math problem. Intimacy is created through the shared experience of values and vulnerabilities. Marlatt et al. describe the relationship through their work on mindfulness-based relapse prevention in the area of addictive behavior. For them, the open, accepting attitude of the therapist is key, and provides a contrast with the more judgmental attitude found in a "tough love" approach or in Alcoholics Anonymous.

Safran and Reading assert that one of the major changes in recent times in psychoanalytic circles is the understanding that therapists are not mere spectators but rather engaged participants, such that therapist and client co-create the relational patterns in the therapeutic encounter. Mindfulness of these relational patterns is key to a successful outcome and should be examined collaboratively by the therapist and the client in a feedback loop that they call metacommunication. Mishka Lysack offers the insight that mindfulness in the context of family therapy involves the co-creation of a cooperative, open, dialogic space—a mindfulness of connectedness that is constructed in an ongoing way throughout the therapy process.

6 Mindfulness, Values, and Therapeutic Relationship in Acceptance and Commitment Therapy

KELLY G. WILSON
EMILY K. SANDOZ

At the still point of the turning world. Neither flesh nor fleshless;
Neither from nor towards; at the still point there the dance is,
But neither arrest nor movement. And do not call it fixity,
Where past and future are gathered. Neither from nor towards,
Neither ascent nor decline. Except for the point, the still point,
There would be no dance and only the dance.
—T. S. ELIOT, "Burnt Norton" (1935)

In this chapter, we describe mindfulness processes in acceptance and commitment therapy (ACT) (said as a word, not as an acronym) (Hayes et al., 1999) as they apply to both the therapist and client. We describe ways in which mindfulness and values work in ACT[1] combine to generate a potent therapeutic relationship. The chapter focuses on ways of relating, one human being to another, that foster a powerful working alliance and make valued living a shared creative act in the here and now. What follows should not be considered a comprehensive treatment of the ACT model. For a broader overview of ACT, including the ways in which these components fit into the treatment approach as a whole, the reader is directed to more comprehensive treatments of ACT (e.g., Hayes, Strosahl, & Wilson, 1999; Hayes & Strosahl, 2004).

In order to understand the centrality of mindfulness processes in ACT, one must see the way the client regards his or her own difficulties. There is little present-moment focus and little acceptance. Likewise, to understand the importance and quality of the therapeutic relationship in ACT, it is important to first understand the orientation to relationship the client brings to therapy. The client comes to therapy with a problem and relates to the therapist as the problem solver. The client views his or her suffering as an adversary and the therapist as an ally in the battle.

The most common explicit purpose of psychotherapy is to alleviate some set of signs and symptoms. If it has gone on long enough, our clients begin to lose themselves in their struggle with sadness, anxiety, and fear. As therapists, we listen hard to these struggles. We listen slowly. We listen carefully. We ask our clients to close their eyes and walk us slowly, step by step, breath by breath, through a very hard day. We listen in a way that allows us to feel their feet as they touch the floor, to see the rain spattered window as they look out at the world. We listen in a way that allows us to put our hands on the grit and grain of our clients' suffering.

Why? Because wherever we see such a long, hard slog, we see an equally potent life looking for a way to unfold. And, we wonder—first to ourselves, and then out loud—what would that person do were the struggle to cease? What would occupy the sweet and sad corners of that life? Would they sing out loud? Would they learn to dance the mambo? Would they buy flowers for their spouse for no reason at all? Would they march for peace or take a quiet walk in the woods? It is in this very slow, deliberate listening and wondering that the beginnings of a particular kind of therapeutic relationship are born.

THE PROBLEM OF SUFFERING

The persistence and ubiquity of human suffering are astonishing. While individual disorders are often quite rare, it is only the carving of human suffering into hundreds of categories and subcategories (American Psychiatric Association, 2000) that makes it so. When we set aside for a moment the categories, many of which are of dubious validity (Follette & Houts, 1996), we see quite a different picture. In a telling prevalence study, Kessler and colleagues (1994) found that nearly a third of their community sample could have been diagnosed with a DSM Axis I disorder at some point within a mere 1-year time period.

Depression, anxiety, and myriad other forms of human suffering present themselves as problems to be solved in much the same way as getting the car repaired, cleaning a dirty floor, or balancing the checkbook. Humans are problem solvers. Wherever we go we find problems to solve. As therapists, we are often swept up, without questioning, in the client's problem-solving agenda.

THE PROBLEM OF PROBLEM SOLVING

Mindfulness meditation is a marvelous way to see the ubiquity of human problem solving—the complement to the ubiquity of suffering. Give a human an altogether simple thing to do: sit on a cushion and count breaths to 10, then start over. The very first thing we find is a problem. "Ouch, my knee hurts a little." We adjust the knee and it feels better. "Ahhh." Then we notice our back hurts, so we sit up a little. And, again, "ahhhh." Then we notice our mind wandering and remember that we are supposed to be observing our breath, and so we solve the wandering-mind problem. And the next problem comes up, and is solved. And the next, and the next, ad infinitum.

There is a marvelous thing that happens, however, when we let go of problem solving for just a little while. If we gently let go of each problem as it arises and sit at that still point between action and nonaction, the world fills in around us—lush, detailed, abundant, and rich. Oddly, though problems do not go away (the knee still aches, there is still the laundry to be done), we feel a bit freer. Problem solving seems so wholly sensible. It works in so many places in life. It seems, however, there are other areas of living where this problem solving approach falls short.

In some respects, ACT can be thought of as a method of teaching people to let go of wholly sensible attempts to solve the fundamental problem of human suffering. Typically clients come to therapy with a problem and a plan. The problem is some set of symptoms. The plan is to first solve the problem, and then to live life as they would choose. In ACT, we take an approach that is not anti-problem solving, but assumes that human problem solving persistently drifts from domains of living where problem solving is effective into areas where problem solving is ineffective and at times even destructive.

ACT asks questions of the client. What if problem solving 24 hours a day is not the best way to live? What if problem solving 24 hours a day is not even the best way to problem solve? What if letting go of problem solving and, instead, making contact with exactly where we are at given moment, sitting at that still point, can provide a way to move forward into a life experienced as lush, detailed, abundant, and rich—a life in which we feel freer somehow to move in the direction of things we value?

VALUES AND COMMITMENT IN ACT

The primary purpose of ACT is to embrace necessary suffering in order to increase one's ability to engage in valued living (Strosahl, Hayes, & Wilson, 2004). In ACT, values are defined as a special class of reinforcers that are verbally constructed, dynamic, ongoing patterns of activity for which the predominant reinforcer is intrinsic in the valued behavioral pattern itself (Wilson, Sandoz, Kitchens, & Roberts, 2008). Being a good parent may produce outcomes for our children, such academic and social success. However, even when particular outcomes do not occur, parenting remains important to us. Values are, instead, a chosen direction in which an individual can always move, no matter what milestones are reached.

Likewise, commitment in ACT is not a promise that is made once and that is assumed to organize behavior forever. Commitment involves returning again and again to movement in a valued direction. This is similar to a breathing meditation, in that to meditate is not to notice one's breath without interruption. Interruption is the natural state of affairs. To meditate is to return to the breath each time an interruption is noticed. Similarly, commitment in ACT refers to letting go of interruptions in valued living, and to that gentle turn back toward the chosen value.

Challenges to Work on Values and Commitment

One of the first steps in values and commitment work is for the therapist and client to come to a shared sense of the values that will direct the work in therapy. The integration of values work into therapy can be challenging, as contact with values necessarily involves contact with vulnerabilities. Values and vulnerabilities are poured from the same vessel. When we know what a person values, we know also what can hurt them. This vulnerability, and its associated value, is usually protected by a well-practiced repertoire of defense. While the form of this defensive repertoire varies, the function is to protect what the individual holds dear. From an ACT perspective, obstacles to valued living are found in failures in present-moment processes, avoidance, cognitive fusion, and attachment to limiting self-conceptualization.

Present-Moment Focus and Values

Clients often have trouble contacting values in the present moment. Worry and rumination are the most frequent forms. For example, a woman who values intimate relationships may be so busy ruminating over her behavior in a past relationship or worrying over a future relationship that she fails to pursue any relationship in the here and now.

Fusion and Values

In addition, because values are verbally constructed, individuals may exhibit a particular kind of rigidity referred to in ACT as *cognitive fusion*. Taking the example above, genuinely intimate relations require flexibility and accommodation. Fusion with an idealized relationship can interfere with needed flexibility and ultimately with good functioning in a relationship.

Experiential Avoidance and Values

Also, individuals may exhibit experiential avoidance related to values. A divorced father may find his thoughts of displacement as a parent or memories of his behavior that led to the divorce so aversive that he neglects commitments to the value of parenting. Avoiding these aspects of experience often produce short term relief, but long-term costs.

Limitations of Conceptualized Self and Values

Finally, individuals may have difficulty experiencing themselves as someone who is free to choose and pursue a direction in life. Sometimes individuals struggle to reconcile what they value with "who they are." For example, an older individual who values education may fail to return to school because of attachment to the thought that he or she is "too old" or "too stupid" to learn anything new.

THERAPIST BEHAVIOR AND THE QUALITY
OF THE THERAPEUTIC RELATIONSHIP

Working with values can easily degenerate into navigating problems with the conceptualized past or future, fusion with conceptualized values, values-related experiential avoidance, and limiting self-conceptualization. It is part of the human condition to be problem solvers, and this is no less true of therapists than it is of clients. When presented with a barrage of problems, therapists often feel compelled to dig in and start problem solving. However, this pattern of interaction fosters a therapeutic relationship in which the therapist is whole and competent and the client has (and is) a problem to be solved. The questions ACT asks our clients are appropriate for us as therapists also. What if persistent problem solving is not the best way to help our clients to live? What if persistent problem solving is not even the best way to help our clients to problem solve? What if our readiness to take on the role of the problem solver in the relationship undermines a potentially more powerful therapeutic relationship?

On Math Problems and Sunsets

We often ask therapists interacting with their most intractable clients, "Are your clients math problems or sunsets? Are they problems to be solved or are they sunsets to be appreciated?" Mindful interactions around valued domains can precipitate a strikingly intimate therapeutic relationship. These interactions do not make all problems go away. But, as humans, problems compel us and they compel our clients. And, in that compulsion to problem solve, sunsets are missed along with possibilities for rich experience—both in life and in the therapeutic interaction. In letting go, even momentarily, of problem solving, possibilities emerge and, paradoxically, change becomes possible at just the moment we let go of change as a *necessity*.

ACT AND THE THERAPEUTIC RELATIONSHIP

Therapists from vastly different theoretical orientations note the importance of the therapeutic relationship, making it the "quintessential integrative variable" (Wolfe & Goldfried, 1988, p. 449). There is a quality of relationship that is apparent to the therapist, the client, and even nonparticipant observers, and that consistently predicts positive outcomes in therapy (see Martin, Garske, & Davis, 2000 for a brief review). A progressive science of clinical psychology necessitates specifying means by which such a relationship can be facilitated.

FACILITATING THE THERAPEUTIC RELATIONSHIP

Therapist Values and Vulnerabilities

We believe that values and vulnerabilities are central to facilitating an intimate working relationship. If we look at our own most intimate relationships, what we find is shared knowledge of values and vulnerabilities. People with whom we feel most intimate are those who know both what we care most about and what we most fear. This is contrary to the common idea that values and vulnerabilities *follow* the establishment of intimacy. We believe that deliberate, mindful insertion of therapist values and vulnerabilities into the therapeutic interaction can produce a potent connection between client and therapist.

Clients come into therapy bearing considerable vulnerability. This creates an imbalance in the relationship. Genuine intimacy in a relationship involves two people standing on shared ground. Thus, the therapist begins by placing his or her own values and vulnerability into the interaction. These values, in so far as they are relevant to treatment, are to be found in the therapist's genuine concern for the client's ability to live a life in which they feel freer to pursue their values. The therapist will not be able to make intimate contact with the client's values and vulnerabilities without the client's help. Therein lies the therapist's vulnerability. The therapist is powerless to move forward without access that only the client can give. A deliberate mindful expression of both this value and vulnerability works to level the ground upon which the therapist and client stand. To do so, we slow the pace of conversation, lean forward, and give direct expression to our value and our vulnerability:

> "I have lots of skills and lots of training. But, none of these will be any help to me without something only you can offer. In order for me to be useful to you, I need you to help me to feel what the world feels like from inside your skin. I have listened to your difficulties, and have heard something of the things you feel are missing in your life. I can sense a longing you feel for something more in life—something richer, freer. I would like to be an agent of that. It would mean a lot to me to be your instrument. Would you help me to see the world through your eyes, to feel what you feel? Would you help me to be your instrument?"

An additional critical component in building the therapeutic relationship is contained in the conclusion in the transcript above. Permission to make close experiential contact with the client's vulnerabilities is sought. The request makes clear the therapist's values and vulnerabilities and also puts the client in control. All the creatures of the earth prefer difficult things they can predict and or control over difficult things that they can neither predict nor control (see Wilson & Murrell, 2004, for fuller discussion). To allow clients to set the pace in this way means relating to them in a way that is both respectful and sensitive. As a general rule, a therapist can never ask permission too intently or too often. Simply adding "Would you be willing to try this?" or "Please help me to really get this" is often enough to extend the therapeutic contract.

Bringing Mindfulness Processes to the Therapeutic Relationship

In the preceding sections on therapeutic relationship, we allude to a quality of interaction that is at least as important as the content. We adopt a deliberate, focused listening and speaking, which make it possible to approach the sensitive area of values and vulnerabilities in alliance and with permission. In training we often refer to the qualities of the interaction as *mindfulness for two.*

Mindfulness has been defined in a number of ways from a number of different perspectives, specifying different processes, outcomes, and even interventions (e.g., Bishop et al., 2004; Dimidjian & Linehan, 2003; Kabat-Zinn, 1994; Langer, 2000; Marlatt & Kristeller, 1999; and see Hick, Chapter 1, this volume). For the purposes of this paper, we focus on mindfulness as a process. The ACT model of psychological health specifies a total of six interrelated processes. In addition to values and committed action, the four remaining component processes (being present, acceptance, defusion, and transcendent sense of self) make up a way of being that contains many of the elements of what is commonly referred to as mindfulness (see Fletcher & Hayes, 2005).

Present-Moment Processes

Present-moment processes refer to the capacity to bring attention to bear in a flexible and focused way in the present moment. Flexibility, within this definition, distinguishes this process from rigidly fixed attention such as might be seen in video game play. Focus distinguishes this process from distractibility, such as might be seen when various events in turn capture attention absent a deliberate quality of attention.

Acceptance

Acceptance involves an intentional openness to one's experience without attempting to diminish or alter its frequency, form, or intensity. Acceptance is not equivalent to liking or wanting. Experiencing pain or discomfort is not, in and of itself, seen as virtuous. However, being willing to experience pain or discomfort, without defense, can make valued living possible.

Defusion

Cognitive defusion is relating to events, including aspects of private experience, in such a way as to increase flexibility. Fusion is viewed as a problem to the extent that it interferes with valued living. For example, the thought "I cannot stand this panic attack" may capture attention and awareness in such a way as to narrow behavior and reduce capacity for valued living. ACT does not intervene on the validity of the thought, as might be done in traditional cognitive therapy. Instead, acceptance and openness to thoughts, both positive and negative, is fostered through predominantly experiential, rather than logical, interventions.

Transcendent Sense of Self

From a behavioral perspective, "self" is not thing-like (Hayes, 1984; Skinner, 1974). Instead, self is considered an ongoing stream of behavior born in, and being dynamically shaped by, that crucible of questions the answers to which begin with "I." A narrow focus on difficult content has the potential to narrow the breadth of the experience of self. In order to discriminate a sense of self distinct from the contents of consciousness, multiple exemplars are required. To the extent that our clients are engaged in a broad set of questions, in a slow and deliberate fashion, they are more likely to notice the "I" that notices. Focus on difficulties alone carries the risk of fostering fusion of self with difficulties (i.e., I = depressed, I = anxious). In the service of noticing this transcendent sense of self, we bring our attention to bear in therapy on both sweet and sad moments. We move with flexibility and deliberate pacing among questions about values, vulnerabilities, and struggles.

Effects of Therapist Mindfulness

Therapists who are themselves engaging in these processes are more sensitive to subtle changes in the client's behavior. If therapists can discriminate subtle shifts in the stream of client behavior, they can then teach those discriminations to the client. Also, the therapist who is exhibiting mindfulness is modeling the very behaviors or she is hoping to elicit in the client. Thus, therapist mindfulness creates a context in which client mindfulness is more likely to emerge.

VALUES AND THE MINDFUL RELATIONSHIP

The Sweet-Spot Exercise

A relatively simple method of facilitating contact with client values has been developed in the form of an experiential exercise known as the "Sweet Spot" (Wilson, 2005). In the Sweet-Spot Exercise, the client expresses to the therapist a moment in his or her life that was sweet, and the therapist appreciates the sweetness in that moment. The therapist might introduce the exercise by saying something like the following:

> "You've told me of some of your struggles and I think that I am starting to understand what brought you here. What I'd really like to get right now, at this moment, is where you've found sweetness in your life. I'm wondering if you would call to mind a moment when you felt really alive, when the struggle that has had its grip on you just fell away for a moment—a moment completely without effort, when you knew who you were, and where you belonged. It could be something recent or something long past. I'd like you to call to mind just one. It doesn't have to be the most important or the happiest moment. It may be something really simple. You may even find a little bit of sadness there. See if you can just let that be there for just a moment. Just allow yourself to drift back into that moment and just be there briefly, in that moment of sweetness. Do you have it? [Client indicates "yes."] Good. Now I'd like you to linger there just a moment longer and when I say so, I want you to express to me what this moment was like in a way that I will *get* it. I may not *understand* exactly what was happening, how it came about, or why it was important, but as you express, I should be able to *get* that this was a moment of your life that was truly sweet."

The focus of this exercise is client and therapist contact with the client's values. It is not important that the value is named, so long as both the client and the therapist experience it. This is a good exercise for values work early in treatment because it includes very little that would encourage the explaining and evaluation that might go on if you simply asked a client in his or her first session, "So, what do you value?" The exercise sets a tone and pace for the relationship that distinguish it from ordinary social interactions. We use this exercise as an example of how values work can target the mindfulness processes in ACT, and how doing so fosters a close working alliance.

Valued Living and Present-Moment Processes

Certain qualities of values and commitment interventions can help to facilitate contact with the present moment during the work. Applying them specifically to the Sweet-Spot Exercise, a therapist might precede the exercise with an eyes-closed noticing exercise, where the client is guided in noticing sensations (sounds, temperature, bodily sensations, and so on) and moves to a mindfulness exercise targeting the Sweet Spot. Throughout, the therapist should use a slow, steady, and deliberate tone and cadence in speaking, using variability to draw the client's attention to particulars in the present moment. The therapist's voice is the primary instrument in setting the pace of the mindful interaction that will follow. As a general rule, it is much more likely a therapist will move too quickly through the exercise than too slowly. Pauses should be inserted frequently throughout. A good way for therapists to pace themselves is by pausing to follow each instruction they give the client.

"I'll start by asking you to allow yourself to sit in a way that will be comfortable to sit—with your feet on the ground, hands in your lap. And, I'll ask you to just gently, gently let your eyes go closed. I'd like you to begin by noticing the different sounds in the room. If you could imagine that you have a sort of checklist, I'd like you to just notice, beginning with the most prominent sounds, just notice them and imagine that you check them off the list. See if you can listen for smaller, more subtle sounds. You might hear the sounds of vehicles outside, the murmur of people speaking in other rooms. And, breathe. Begin to draw your attention to your own body. Begin to notice places where your body makes contact with the floor and the chair. And, breathe. Notice especially the little places where you can feel the transition in that contact. Notice the very edges of the place on your back that are touching the chair. See if in your mind's eye you can trace that margin. See if you can begin to notice the smallest details in sensation that tell you this part is touching and that is not. And, breathe.

"Now, I'd like you to imagine that in front of you there is a file cabinet. In the file cabinet let there be photographs. Imagine that you open the drawer and reach in and withdraw a picture of you during that sweet moment. And, if there is not a picture there, just let one materialize. Let yourself draw that picture up from the file cabinet and feel it in your hands. Let yourself notice the sensations in your fingertips as you gently hold the photo. Let yourself look into that face of yours in that picture and let yourself notice the details surrounding you. Let yourself see your own face—the cut of your hair, the set of your jaw, the look in your eyes. And now, I want you to imagine that your awareness is some sort of liquid that could be poured into that *you* in that picture. So, imagine that your awareness is beginning to pour into the skin of that you *in that very moment*. See if you can let yourself emerge in that place at that particular moment. Imagine opening your eyes in that place. Let yourself see what you see there. Let yourself notice the sensations that you feel on your own skin in that sweet place. If you are outdoors perhaps you feel a slight breeze. If you're with someone you might feel the warmth of their skin against you, the scent of their hair. Let it be as if you could just breathe that moment in and out. Let yourself feel the life in that moment. As if each breath filled you with that sweetness. Let it be as if every cell in your body can feel what it is to be in that place. Just take a moment to luxuriate in that presence. And now, I'm going to ask you to gently, gently let your eyes open. I don't want you to speak yet. Let yourself look into my eyes and let yourself notice that there is a person sitting right here. Here I am, a person who has known sweetness too. I want to just gently let your sweet moment fill you—slowly, slowly like some liquid. And, when you're ready I want you to gently begin to speak and give expression to that sweetness. Go gently as if you were walking through a forest. If you walk very quietly, you might see things that you would miss if you hurried. So, in the gentlest way you can, let that sweet moment be expressed. Let me hear, feel, see that sweet moment."

The expression of sweetness and, just as important, the therapist's appreciation will be enhanced if this brief mindfulness exercise precedes expression and appreciation. While the client is expressing, the therapist should focus on the client's presentation like a meditation, noticing the sounds of the words and the qualities of the experience that the client is conveying. The mindful, attentive quality of this interaction will precipitate strong connection between therapist and client.

This is an exercise in expression and appreciation, not explaining and understanding. Metaphorically, one could explain and/or understand a sunset, including the physics of the refraction of light through water particles in the atmosphere. However, there might also be value in a simple act of appreciation. Thus, the therapist should ask clients in advance to very deliberately slow their pace of speech as they express— savoring each word and sensation.

During this exercise, clients will often lose the present moment-focus of the interaction. Listen for transitions in the client's pace and pitch of speech, from a lingering, deliberate pace to one with a more conversational quality. When clients speed up, gently coach them to return to a slower pace. Failure to do so will result in a return to more commonplace conversations and to the fruits of those more common conversations.

The coaching of pace should itself be delivered in a gentle, deliberate fashion. Watch also for transitions in therapist responding. If therapists notice themselves analyzing, comparing, evaluating, or attempting to understand they should notice that distraction and gently come back to a simple appreciation of the client's expression. This sort of interaction fosters an intensity and genuineness of communication that forms the basis of a strong therapeutic alliance.

Valued Living and the Transcendent Sense of Self

People do not contact values through the stories they have about themselves (i.e., fusion with self-as-content). Any intervention that encourages flexible, present moment focused interaction with the self beyond conceptualizations should facilitate this contact. Applied specifically to the Sweet-Spot Exercise, several modifications can enhance the emergence of this transcendent sense of self. When the client is expressing, the therapist might stay focused on the client's eyes and resist the urge to convey understanding by nodding, asking questions, and so on. It is not so much the conveyance of understanding that is the concern, but the ways that these subtle social cues lead us back to the realm of day-to-day conversation, and away from this mindfulness exercise for two. We manage impressions of ourselves a good deal in ordinary conversation. The exercise is designed to detune impression management and create a context for more of a person-to-person interaction. Provide clients with a warning beforehand that you might stop them before they have finished speaking and allow for some period of time where their eyes continue to express the sweetness of that moment—even without words. During the exercise, when pace escalates say something like:

"Allow yourself to fall silent for just a minute. I don't want you to begin speaking again until I tell you to. And while you are silent, I want you to continue expressing, but with only your eyes. See if you can just let your experience, your moment of sweetness, pour out of you like water."

This exercise is often intense and tends to foster an experience of "seeing" and of being "seen," for both the client and the therapist. In addition, the therapist might ask the client to notice the "I" that was there, in that moment of sweetness, that has always been there, and that they still carry with them now (the therapist, meanwhile, noticing the same in his or her own experience). Finally, the therapist might reflect on his or her experience with the client, for example:

"Just then, while you were speaking, something happened. I noticed all the stories you have about you fell away for a second and for a moment I saw just you. Not the 'you' who has to be smart or funny or strong or good, but in your eyes for just a moment, you were just . . . you."

There is an assumption built into this exercise that relationship between two individuals (including therapist and client) is enhanced by both individuals being fully present as persons. When therapists and clients are excessively attached to their respective roles, and what they "should" look like in the therapeutic interaction, they can sometimes miss one another as persons. The exercise is designed to erode the separation that roles sometimes impose.

Valued Living and Acceptance

When values are contacted, all the "have-to's" of daily existence fall away, and the client is free to be, without changing his or her experience at all. Certain qualities of values and commitment interventions can help to facilitate this kind of acceptance during the work. Any intervention that involves saying yes to painful experiences related to values should make avoidance less likely. For example, often the Sweet Spot will be bittersweet, involving some sorrow or remorse. The therapist may call attention to this sorrow specifically during the exercise:

"And now, in the middle of all that sweetness, I want you to notice if there isn't just a kernel of sorrow there. Just a little piece of longing that shows up there all mixed in with that joy. I want you to see if you can notice the edges of that sorrow, where you feel it in your body. Now I want you to slowly, slowly breathe in that sorrow as if it were air. See if, just for a moment, you can let go of managing and just let yourself breathe the sweet and sad gently, gently in and out."

Valued Living and Defusion

Valued living is not a formally defined, inflexible pattern of activity. Rather, it is a dynamic stream of activity. Any intervention that promotes flexible interaction with verbal constructions of the value should make fusion less likely. For example after the client has expressed, the therapist may repeat back words that provoked his or her own responding to "shoulds" or "needs." The therapist assumes that those that provoked him or her may also be likely to provoke the client.

> "Now I'm going to say back to you some of the words I really felt when you spoke, and I'd like you to just notice what shows up for you as you hear these words.
>
>   "Daughter . . .
>   "Happy . . .
>   "Disappointment . . .
>   "Love . . . "

The therapist might then ask the client what he or she noticed—all the while retaining the mindful pace of the conversation. The therapist should repeat these words slowly and deliberately, savoring the sound of the words. In doing so, the richness of the word may begin to emerge, the sound of the word, thoughts, memories, and emotions provoked— all gently noticed and released in turn. Again, the therapist should be watchful for changes in the pace and pitch of the client's speech. When specific words provoke a call to action, the therapist might return to the expression part of the exercise, repeating these words individually and pausing, asking the client to notice reactions and express a felt sense of those to the therapist. It is important that this interaction not devolve into problem solving. The therapist should actively coach gentle expression and appreciation.

Moving among Processes

As mentioned previously, these processes are interdependent. This is reflected in the way they are trained as well. As a matter of principle, mindfulness processes are thought to undermine cognitive fusion and nonacceptance that obstruct valued living. Cognitive fusion and nonacceptance are characterized by a narrowness and inflexibility in behavior. Use of these methods is appropriate when we see the emergence of narrowness and inflexibility in behavior, particularly when that inflexibility impacts valued living. When we see behavioral flexibility emerge, more instrumental interventions involving values and committed action are appropriate. Because fusion and nonacceptance are seen as pervasive in the human condition, therapy typically involves moving between mindfulness and acceptance processes on the one hand, and committed action and behavior change processes on the other.

CONCLUSION

In the preceding sections, we have presented a rationale and structure for building the mindful therapeutic relationship within the ACT model. In doing so, we have reflected on the connection between core ACT processes and the building of that relationship. We do so because, within the ACT model, it doesn't make sense to speak of the therapeutic relationship independent of these processes.

The general therapeutic model of ACT has produced good preliminary data on a wide variety of outcomes including psychotic disorders (Bach & Hayes, 2002; Gaudiano & Herbert, 2006), chronic pain and stress (Bond & Bunce, 2000; Dahl, Wilson, & Nilsson, 2004; McCracken, Vowles, & Eccleston, in press), and epilepsy (Dahl & Lundgren, 2005). Further, the data suggest that across client difficulties, settings, and modes of delivery, positive outcomes of ACT are mediated by improvements in particular facets of mindfulness, such as acceptance and defusion (see Hayes, Luoma, Bond, Masuda, & Lillis, 2006, for a review).

However, because outcome and process research in ACT is in its infancy, the interventions described in this chapter should be viewed as suggestions for clinical action and as a call for basic research into the psychological processes described here. Assertions in this chapter regarding methods for fostering a strong therapeutic alliance are extrapolated from theory and from a body of basic and applied evidence. Even though the general ACT model appears robust, we ought not conclude that all the processes described in the theory are necessary for preferred outcomes to occur. In a certain very important sense, all scientific theories are wrong (Hayes, 2007). The difference between old and new theories is that we know *how* the old theories are wrong.

We likewise call for basic research to expand our understanding of the use of mindfulness in therapy more generally. Although the traditions from which mindfulness has been drawn are quite old, and not without demonstrated potency, the science of mindfulness is in the earliest stages. It is likely that the theories that gave brought us to this stage will not take us to the next—at least not in their current form. However, with persistent interest in mindfulness and dedication to empirical principles, the continued scientific progress into the applications of mindfulness in therapy is as promising as it is new.

REFERENCES

American Psychiatric Association. (2000). *Diagnostic and statistical manual of mental disorders* (4th ed., text rev.). Washington, DC: Author.

Bach, P., & Hayes, S. C. (2002). The use of acceptance and commitment therapy to prevent the rehospitalization of psychotic patients: A randomized controlled trial. *Journal of Consulting and Clinical Psychology, 70,* 1129–1139.

Bishop, S. R., Lau, M., Shapiro, S., Carlson, L., Anderson, N. D. Carmody, J., et al. (2004) Mindfulness: A proposed operational definition. *Clinical Psychology: Science and Practice, 11*(3), 230–241.

Bond, F. W., & Bunce, D. (2000). Outcomes and mediators of change in emotion-focused and problem-focused worksite stress management interventions. *Journal of Occupational Health Psychology, 5,* 156–163.

Dahl, J., & Lundgren, T. (2005). Behavior analysis of epilepsy: Conditioning mechanisms, behavior technology and the contribution of ACT. *Behavior Analyst Today, 6,* 191–202.

Dahl, J., Wilson, K. G., & Nilsson, A. (2004). Acceptance and commitment therapy and the treatment of persons at risk for long-term disability resulting from stress and pain symptoms: A preliminary randomized trial. *Behavior Therapy, 35,* 785–801.

Dimidjian, S. D., & Linehan, M. M. (2003). Mindfulness practice. In W. O'Donohue, J. Fisher, & S. Hayes (Eds.), *Cognitive behavior therapy: Applying empirically supported techniques in your practice* (pp. 229–237). New York: Wiley.

Fletcher, L., & Hayes, S. C. (2005). Relational frame theory, acceptance and commitment therapy, and a functional analytic definition of mindfulness. *Journal of Rational Emotive and Cognitive Behavioral Therapy, 23,* 315–336.

Follette, W. C., & Houts, A. C. (1996). Models of scientific progress and the role of theory in taxonomy development: A case study of the DSM. *Journal of Consulting and Clinical Psychology, 64,* 1120–1132.

Gaudiano, B. A., & Herbert, J. D. (2006). Acute treatment of inpatients with psychotic symptoms using acceptance and commitment therapy. *Behaviour Research and Therapy, 44,* 415–437.

Hayes, S. C. (1984). Making sense of spirituality. *Behaviorism, 12,* 99–110.

Hayes, S. C. (2007, July). *The state of the evidence in acceptance and commitment therapy.* Paper presented at the Third Summer Institute for ACT, RFT, and Contextual Behavioral Science, Houston, TX.

Hayes, S. C., Luoma, J., Bond, F., Masuda, A., and Lillis, J. (2006). Acceptance and commitment therapy: Model, processes, and outcomes. *Behaviour Research and Therapy, 44,* 1–25.

Hayes, S. C., Strosahl, K., & Wilson, K. G. (1999). *Acceptance and commitment therapy: An experiential approach to behavior change.* New York: Guilford Press.

Hayes, S. C., & Strosahl, K. D. (2004). *A practical guide to acceptance and commitment therapy.* New York: Springer-Verlag.

Kabat-Zinn, J. (1994). *Wherever you go there you are: Mindfulness meditation in everyday life.* New York: Hyperion.

Kessler, R. C., McGonagle, K. A., Zhao, S., Nelson, C. B., Hughes, M., Eshleman, S., et al. (1994). Lifetime and 12-month prevalence of DSM-III-R psychiatric disorders in the United States: Results from the National Comorbidity Study. *Archives of General Psychiatry, 51,* 8–19.

Langer, E. J. (2000). Mindful learning. *Current Directions in Psychological Science, 9,* 220–223.

Marlatt, G. A., & Kristeller, J. L. (1999). Mindfulness and meditation. In W. R. Miller (Ed.), *Integrating spirituality into treatment* (pp. 67–84). Washington, DC: American Psychological Association.

Martin, D. J., Garske, J. P., & Davis, M. K. (2000). Relation of the therapeutic alliance with outcome and other variables: A meta-analytic review. *Journal of Consulting and Clinical Psychology, 68,* 438–450.

McCracken, L. M., Vowles, K. E., & Eccleston, C. (2005). Acceptance-based treatment for persons with complex, long-standing chronic pain: A preliminary analysis of treatment outcome in comparison to a waiting phase. *Behavior Research and Therapy, 43,* 1335–1346.

Skinner, B. F. (1974). *About behaviorism.* New York: Knopf.

Strosahl, K., Hayes, S. C., & Wilson, K. G. (2004). An acceptance and commitment therapy primer: Core therapy processes, intervention strategies, and therapist competencies. In S. C. Hayes & K. Strosahl (Eds.), *A practical guide to acceptance and commitment therapy* (pp. 31–58). New York: Springer Press.

Wilson, K. G. (July, 2005). *Eroding the illusion of separation: The interplay of core ACT processes in group training.* Paper presented at the 2005 ACT/RFT Summer Institute II, LaSalle University, Philadelphia.

Wilson, K. G., & Murrell, A. R. (2004). Values work in acceptance and commitment therapy: Setting a course for behavioral treatment. In S. C. Hayes, V. M. Follette, & M. Linehan (Eds.), *Mindfulness and acceptance: Expanding the cognitive-behavioral tradition* (pp. 120–151). New York: Guilford Press.

Wilson, K. G., Sandoz, E. K., Kitchens, J., & Roberts, M. E. (2008). *The Valued Living Questionnaire: Defining and measuring valued action within a behavioral framework.* Manuscript submitted for publication.

Wolfe, B. E., & Goldfried, M. R. (1988). Research on psychotherapy integration: Recommendations and conclusions from an NIMH workshop. *Journal of Consulting and Clinical Psychology, 56,* 448–451.

7 Mindfulness-Based Relapse Prevention for Substance Abusers

*Therapist Training
and Therapeutic Relationships*

G. ALAN MARLATT
SARAH BOWEN
NEHA CHAWLA
KATIE WITKIEWITZ

Struggling with the addicted mind is not unique to individuals with substance abuse disorders. The desire to "self-medicate" is common to all human beings, whether manifested in drug and alcohol use, overeating, sexual practices, work habits, or a pervasive need to stay occupied in service of avoiding discomfort. Mindfulness practice presents a radically different approach to working with discomfort: cultivating a curiosity and willingness to "lean in" to the experience, rather than to "fix" or avoid it. Modeling of such a stance is critical for individuals beginning to adopt a more mindful and accepting attitude. In mindfulness-based relapse prevention (MBRP; Witkiewitz, Marlatt, & Walker, 2005), as in many of the mindfulness- or acceptance-based therapies, one of the key roles of therapists is an embodiment of this stance, both in their own personal practices and approach to experience, and in the style with which they interact with clients. The therapeutic relationship developed in the environment of an MBRP course can serve as a model of a nonjudgmental and compassionate approach for working with the craving, attachment, and discomfort so often experienced by clients in recovery. The therapist's personal mindfulness practice, which fosters a deeper understanding of these principles, is paramount to the formation of such a relationship.

The current chapter begins by discussing the roots and foundations of MBRP, a new behavioral treatment that integrates traditional cognitive-behavioral relapse prevention (RP; Marlatt & Gordon, 1985) techniques with mindfulness meditation for treatment of substance use disorders. The chapter describes development, training, and implementation of the MBRP protocol, and the role of both therapists' and clients' mindfulness practice in enhancing group cohesion and alliance. Particular focus is given to factors that enhance the therapeutic relationship. Further, aspects of the relationship that are unique to this intervention are highlighted, as well as differences between fundamental approaches of MBRP and more traditional approaches to substance abuse treatment.

At the root of MBRP is the practice of mindfulness meditation, based on the traditional Buddhist practice of *vipassana*, which literally translates as "seeing things as they really are." The practice begins with observation of the breath and expands to include awareness of bodily sensations, thoughts, emotional states, and all aspects of current experience. Mindfulness practitioners are taught to approach their experience in a nonjudgmental fashion, while observing the pulls of attachment and aversion (Hart, 1987). While traditional courses in *vipassana* meditation require up to ten days of highly intensive training in a residential setting, with students meditating for up to 10 hours a day, several recently developed therapies integrate the core practices and principles of *vipassana* into cognitive-behavioral structures more familiar to Western clinicians and clientele.

MBRP is largely based on the practices and structure of mindfulness-based stress reduction for chronic pain (MBSR; Kabat-Zinn, 1982, 1990) and mindfulness-based cognitive therapy for depression (MBCT; Segal, Teasdale, & Williams, 2002; Teasdale, Segal, & Williams, 1995), similarly using a secularized approach to mindfulness practice in combination with techniques based on cognitive-behavioral therapy (CBT). Corresponding in structure, MBRP consists of eight 2-hour sessions delivered in group format over the course of 8 weeks. It has been proposed that in order for mindfulness techniques to be most effective, certain components should be tailored to the particular needs of the population (Teasdale, Segal, & Williams, 2003). MBRP incorporates exercises, meditations, and homework activities specifically tailored to recognizing and coping with craving, triggers, and high-risk situations for substance use.

The research literature on treatment of substance dependence includes numerous studies that have described the clinical and cost effectiveness of CBT in the rise of abstinence rates, reduction of drug and alcohol use (Kadden, 2001), and prevention of relapse (Carroll, 1996; Irvin, Bowers, Dunn, & Wang, 1999). Based on the premise that maladaptive substance use is learned behavior, CBT for substance dependence attempts to identify contextual, social, affective, and cognitive precipitants of substance use. Additionally, the treatment aims to improve interpersonal skills and substitute positive life activities for drug use (Marlatt & Donovan, 2005; Marlatt & Gordon, 1985). Relapse prevention, in particular, relies on the initial assessment of potentially high-risk situations for relapse (e.g., environmental stressors, personality characteristics; see Witkiewitz & Marlatt, 2007), monitoring of behavior in high-risk situations, and assessment of lifestyle factors (e.g., lifestyle imbalance) that may increase the probability of encountering high-risk situations (Larimer, Palmer, & Marlatt, 1999).

MBRP: AN OVERVIEW

In the original description of RP (Marlatt & Gordon, 1985), mindfulness meditation was proposed as a means of helping clients achieve lifestyle balance. Today, MBRP has expanded the use of meditation as a means to achieve balance by thoroughly integrating specific RP strategies (Larimer et al., 1999; Marlatt & Donovan, 2005) into a mindfulness-based treatment. As suggested by Breslin, Zack, and McMain (2002), helping clients recognize their emotional and cognitive responses to triggers for substance use interrupts the previously automatic response of using substances. Indeed, neurobiological findings support the hypothesis that meditation enhances awareness and may help individuals generate alternatives to mindless, compulsive behavior. As described by Groves and Farmer (1994), "In the context of addictions, mindfulness might mean becoming aware of triggers for craving . . . and choosing to do something else which might ameliorate or prevent craving, so weakening the habitual response" (p. 189). Mindfulness meditation may disrupt habitual craving responses by providing heightened awareness and even acceptance of the initial craving response, without judgment or reactance.

The goal of MBRP is to develop awareness and acceptance of thoughts, feelings, and sensations through practicing mindfulness, to observe both pleasant and unpleasant experience, and to accept whatever is present without judgment. These practices are combined with traditional relapse prevention techniques for developing effective coping skills, enhancing self-efficacy, and learning to recognize common antecedents of substance use and relapse (e.g., outcome expectancies, the abstinence violation effect, drinking motives, social pressure). Observation and acceptance are both coping strategies (Marlatt, 2002), in which the focus is on acceptance of the present moment and observation of cognitive, sensory, physical, and intuitive experiences, without analyzing, judging, or emotional responding. The focus is not on "doing what's right" or making "good decisions," but rather on a state of "just being" (Segal et al., 2002). Identification of one's individual high-risk situations for relapse remains a central component of the treatment. Clients are trained to recognize early warning signs for relapse and to increase awareness of substance-related cues, such as people and places that have previously been associated with substance use. Mindfulness practice provides clients with a new way of processing situational cues and monitoring reactions to environmental contingencies.

One example of a coping strategy taught in MBRP is a technique called "urge surfing" (Marlatt & Kristeller, 1999). Urge surfing uses the imagery of a wave to help a client gain control over impulses to use drugs or alcohol. The client is first taught to label internal sensations and cognitive preoccupations as urges, and then to foster an attitude of unattached, curious observation of the experience. The technique focuses on identifying and accepting the urge, rather than acting on or attempting to fight it using suppression or avoidance strategies. The curious and accepting attitude taken by facilitators and trainers toward the experiences of participants models this stance. The thoughts, feelings, and sensations experienced by participants are identified simply as arising events, without judgment, evaluation, or attempts to alter and control them. This includes aversive states such as cravings and urges, as well as physical and emotional discomfort. Accepting the occurrence of thoughts and experiences rather than attempting to avoid or suppress them has been shown to be an effective component of mindfulness practice in relation to decreased substance use (Bowen, Witkiewitz, Dillworth, & Marlatt, 2007). In a recent study on the effectiveness of *vipassana* meditation in reducing substance use (see Bowen et al., 2006;

Marlatt et al., 2004), clients reported that "staying in the moment" and being mindful of urges were the most helpful coping strategies.

MBRP may be particularly effective for individuals who are inclined to use substances to ameliorate negative affective states (sometimes in response to craving or other internal or external stimuli). Negative affect has been identified as one of the primary predictors of relapse (Marlatt, 1978; Marlatt & Gordon, 1985; Cummings, Gordon, & Marlatt, 1980), and numerous studies suggest a strong relationship between negative affect and substance use (Shiffman et al., 1996; Witkiewitz & Marlatt, 2004). After repeated experiences of the immediate alleviation of negative affective states through the use of substances, the experience of negative affect can elicit a conditioned response of craving. Meditation provides an opportunity to practice new responses to cues, such as observation and acceptance of experiences, thus replacing the habitual self-medication of negative emotional states with substances.

MBRP: IMPLEMENTATION

Our research group is currently conducting the first feasibility and efficacy trial of MBRP. This trial is composed of three phases: initial development of the MBRP protocol and therapist training, a pilot study, and a main implementation trial. To date, only the pilot phase has been completed. This phase consisted of conducting four gender-segregated groups in conjunction with a private treatment agency. There was no control condition for this phase; the purpose was to provide an opportunity for therapists to practice leading groups, and to incorporate feedback from clients about the content and process of the MBRP groups. The second phase of the study, currently in progress, involves conducting MBRP groups as part of an aftercare program in a community treatment agency. Study participants who are randomly assigned to the control condition continue with their usual aftercare. Groups are mixed gender and consist of 6 to 11 participants. In all phases of the trial, groups meet weekly for 2 hours and are co-led by two therapists. Throughout the first two phases of the study, trainers and therapists learned to acknowledge, with compassion, the therapists' own struggles in maintaining a personal mindfulness practice. It is important for fellow therapists, therapist supervisors, and the research team to uphold the same accepting, nonjudgmental, and compassionate stance toward clients and therapists alike.

THE ROLE OF THE THERAPIST'S PERSONAL PRACTICE
IN THE THERAPEUTIC ALLIANCE

The elemental principles and practices of MBRP are rooted in the basic tenets of Buddhism. Although the treatment does not explicitly reference Buddhism, it remains faithful to the core Buddhist principles regarding the nature of the mind and human suffering. Inherent in these principles is the assumption that human beings universally experience discontent or dissatisfaction, attributable to the nature of the mind itself, which is conditioned to become attached to a world that is impermanent. According to Buddhist philosophy, relief from suffering lies in direct observation of the nature of the mind and the experience of thoughts, sensations, and emotions as impermanent phenomena rather than fixed or permanent states. This allows individuals to respond with awareness rather than react automatically. MBRP is an extension of this theory and practice, tailored to meet the needs of individuals struggling with addiction.

In any therapeutic relationship (see also Lambert & Simon, Chapter 2, this volume), the alliance between clients and therapists is a critical component of the change process, providing a necessary foundation for creating an atmosphere of safety, confidence, and trust. In MBRP, the alliance between the therapists and clients is particularly crucial, as the nonjudgmental curiosity and openness of the therapists toward group members provide a model for clients' development of a mindful, accepting, and compassionate approach to their own experience. The therapists' embodiment of these qualities, and the therapeutic relationship that begins to develop as a result of this approach, is one of the most powerful teaching tools in MBRP.

This nonjudgmental, egalitarian stance may be particularly important for clients who have a history of "tough love" or Higher-Power-focused substance abuse treatments (e.g., 12-step programs such as Alcoholics Anonymous [AA]) and who may have struggled with the evaluative or judgmental nature of these treatments. The MBRP therapist, in contrast, is not only working to develop the alliance with clients but must also take the extra steps of socializing clients to a nonhierarchical, nonstigmatizing, and compassion-focused approach to treatment. For example, throughout the course of the groups, clients often make comments such as "that's because I am an addict" or ask if they will be able to successfully engage in mindfulness meditation exercises because they hold the belief that their brain is different from, and inferior to, a "non-addict's." The therapists repeatedly enforce the equalizing approach of MBRP, wherein the struggles clients are encountering are more about being human than about being an "addict." Therapists reiterate that the experience of craving and the pull to reach for something to ameliorate discomfort is just how the mind works, and that craving and addiction are present in all humans in some form; it is just part of the human experience. Clients are encouraged to treat evaluative and self-judgmental thoughts as "just thoughts" that arise and pass away, rather than as factual truths to be identified with. They are asked to bring the same curiosity and gentleness toward these thoughts and the emotions they may trigger as toward all other experience.

This nonjudgmental therapeutic stance was cultivated from the initial phases of manual development and therapist training. Therapist training began with an intensive two-and-a-half day program, beginning with a basic overview of the theory, history, and design of MBRP. The remainder of the training consisted of meditation and RP skills-based exercises designed to give therapists an experience similar to that of future clients. The trainers alternated between leading exercises and meta-teaching about the process and style of leading the groups.

Throughout the training, concepts behind MBRP were illustrated through experiential exercises wherever possible instead of through didactics, moving through as much of the material in "real time" as possible. The trainees' personal experience and feedback were encouraged. Early in the training, it became clear that the desired dynamic was that of a facilitated group process, rather than a psychoeducational group. Within the MBRP groups, therapists are referred to as facilitators, and clients as group participants.

Throughout the next phase of training, involving weekly group training and practice sessions, therapists were asked to play mock group clients, while other therapists took turns leading the sessions. It quickly became apparent that the experiences in these training groups were likely to bear significant similarity to the experiences of the future clients. Training groups were run with trainees portraying their "real" selves, asking questions about practice, discussing issues in their own practice, and using that material to allow them to practice facilitation skills.

The tenor and format of MBRP therapist training were inspired largely by the structure of MBCT intensive trainings and reflective of the core practices of mindfulness meditation. Embodied in traditional mindfulness practice is a sense of interconnectedness and compassion, both for one's own and for others' experiences. The experience of attachment and suffering is seen as common to all beings, despite evident distinctions in their stories and in the objects of attachment. The trainers hoped to engender, from the very beginnings of development and training, this stance of shared process, cooperation, nonjudgmental openness, and respect. Throughout the training process, which continued for several months, a mindful, nonjudgmental approach was taken toward all experience.

From the beginning phases of therapist recruitment and training, the importance of maintaining a personal practice was emphasized. As with MBCT and MBSR, it was a primary requisite for working on the project that therapists commit to daily personal practice. The practice itself may be viewed at the "true" teacher or guide, and the role of the therapist is one of supporting and encouraging clients while drawing upon their own experience with the practice. Rather than "experts" teaching others what to do, therapists are seen as participants in a common human experience alongside the group members, acting as guides. Although the therapists often differ from clients in manifestations of desire or problematic behaviors, therapists' self-observations and experiences in mindfulness practice are viewed as no different from those of the clients. The sense of shared experience and the importance of therapist engagement in the process are reflected in the feedback received by clients in comments such as "the teachers felt like family."

As the trial began and several teams of therapists began to facilitate MBRP groups, it became apparent that therapists with a strong personal practice were better able to respond to issues and questions that arose both in the training groups and with clients regarding practice. Maintaining a consistent practice allowed them to draw upon their personal experiences in responding to questions and concerns raised by clients regarding challenges such as staying awake during meditations, scheduling time to practice, expecting to attain calm or peaceful states, and working with difficult mental states such as anger and self-criticism. Direct experience with these challenges allowed therapists to respond with a gentleness and honesty that modeled the same attitudes of acceptance and self-compassion that clients were being asked to take toward themselves. They could sincerely acknowledge that setting forty-five minutes aside for meditation practice could seem overwhelming at first, or that sitting through discomfort, boredom, or restlessness was a challenge. Their responses reflected an authenticity that seemed to add to the strength of the alliance with clients. For instance, hearing the therapists disclose that they too struggled with judgmental or distracting thoughts or with challenging emotional states appeared to reassure clients and foster a sense of group cohesion. This is reflected in several comments from clients (i.e., "The explanation that almost everyone has distracting thoughts was very helpful" and "It was good to be able to listen to the struggles of others.")

Many of the practices as well as the style and language used in MBRP are based upon Kabat-Zinn's MBSR protocol (Kabat-Zinn, 1990). Careful use of language during meditations and group discussions further supports a sense of shared experience. Therapists are encouraged to use the word *we* rather than the word *you* to refer to the common group experience and to minimize the distinction between themselves and other members of the group. Therapists are also invited to use the present participle when guiding meditations, to reflect an ongoing and present-centered process of exploration, rather than commands or directives that could potentially create disparity between the experience of the therapist and that of the clients ("allowing" your attention to rest upon the breath vs. "allow" your attention to rest upon the breath).

Numerous in-session exercises encourage clients to be present with painful or uncomfortable emotional experiences. Exercises and meditations are followed by discussion, which often highlights the commonalties between clients' experiences. Therapists acknowledge and accept any observations and challenges that clients share in the group, while encouraging a similar attitude of openness and curiosity toward the thoughts, feelings, and sensations that arise during meditation, without positive or negative valence placed upon any one experience, and without attempts to "fix" discomfort. For example, cravings sometimes arise for clients during the group. Clients are encouraged to stay present with the craving and to bring a gentle and curious awareness to any accompanying thoughts, emotions, and sensations. The therapists might also encourage the other group members to pause and pay attention to any emotions, thoughts, and sensations that may be arising for them in reaction to this. This stance fosters a parallel process between what occurs in the group, that is, a curious and nonjudgmental stance toward clients' experiences, and the aims of personal practice—a compassionate and accepting stance towards one's own experience.

Within this framework, urges and cravings for substances are viewed as just another manifestation of the mind's tendency to cling to pleasant experience and to avoid unpleasant thoughts or sensations. Clients are encouraged to explore cravings as a conglomeration of physical sensations and thoughts, and to experiment with gentle and compassionate observation rather than avoidance or suppression. This may be viewed as novel, uniquely destigmatizing and empowering for individuals who have struggled with addiction and who may have been the subject of repeated judgment and criticism from family, friends, and mental health professionals.

MBRP IN RELATION TO OTHER TREATMENT APPROACHES

As inferred throughout this chapter, techniques used in MBRP integrate several different treatment approaches. In client-centered therapy, developed by Carl Rogers (1959), the therapist adopts an accepting relationship marked by unconditional positive regard, attempting to help the client achieve his or her goals without setting an outside or "top-down" agenda. The style of discussion in MBRP relies heavily on motivational interviewing (MI) techniques, which adopt a similar set of principles, in which the therapist provides active support and collaboration with the client's agenda and treatment goals (Miller & Rollnick, 2002). Here the therapist expresses empathy and compassion toward the client, avoiding argumentation and "rolling with resistance" if it arises in the therapy session. Consistent with the "stages of change" model (Prochaska & DiClemente, 1982) MBRP therapists help work through their clients' ambivalence about change, particularly for those who are in either the precontemplation or contemplation stage and need to work through the pros and cons of making a commitment to an "action plan" designed to achieve treatment goals. Therapists support any efforts made by the client to move toward goal achievement, no matter how small the steps may seem, thereby facilitating self-efficacy.

MBRP therapists also work in congruence with the values incorporated within harm reduction therapy (Marlatt, 1998; Denning, Little, & Glickman, 2003; Tatarsky, 2002). Here the therapist attempts to "meet the clients where they're at" in terms of developing an empathic and nondirective relationship. Rather than setting down fixed rules and regulations, or insisting upon a single treatment goal (e.g., abstinence only), the therapist works on establishing an atmosphere of support and collaboration so as to serve as the client's ally in the process of change. Clients often change their minds, switching between "cutting back" and "giving it up altogether" when it comes to their plans for changing their addictive behavior. Many clients who are unsuccessful in pursuing a moderation or "controlled use" goal will be more motivated to try to give up their alcohol or drug use altogether. On the other hand, if the client is unable or unwilling to pursue total abstinence, or if the client experiences numerous episodes of relapse in abstinence-based programs, a harm-reduction goal may be more successful. For clients who are prone to relapse despite their best efforts to maintain abstinence,

MBRP therapists may draw upon "relapse management" strategies to help them get "back on track" rather than allow them to give up or drop out of treatment (Marlatt & Donovan, 2005). In this approach, the therapist continues to work with the client in developing a positive therapeutic relationship, one based on active partnership and collaboration, as opposed to a more confrontational approach. The relationship between therapist and client is of central importance when considering the various ups and downs experienced by clients in the process of the MBRP course. The therapist stays with the client through setbacks and even major relapses, with the recognition that change is difficult and many clients need positive, compassionate support to counteract a context of negative peer pressure and self-doubt.

The MBRP program differs significantly from other major approaches to changing addictive behavior problems, including both the "moral model" and the "disease model" of addiction (Brickman et al., 1982). In the moral model, the client is assumed to be responsible both for the development of the addiction problem ("It's your fault that you became an alcoholic") and for its eradication. The "War on Drugs" is a prime example of this pejorative approach, in which drug users are punished via severe prison sentences for using or selling illicit substances. Given the recidivism rates (as high as 52.5% of men and 29.7% of women) and relapse rates (as high as 58.5% of men and 42.6% of women) in the 36 months following discharge from prison (Pelissier et al., 2000), it is clear that this approach is an abject failure. It is important to note that prison inmates are rarely offered treatment for their addiction problems (Bender, 2007). Interestingly, several research studies in India and a recent study conducted by our research group (Bowen et al., 2006; Marlatt et al., 2004) have shown mindfulness training is well received by inmates and is related to reductions in drinking and drug use following release from prison.

In the disease model of addiction, clients are told that their problem is due to factors beyond their control, namely biological factors such as genetic predisposition or biological vulnerability to the reinforcing effects of drugs on brain functioning (e.g., Jellinek, 1960). In the traditional model, it is assumed that addiction is a progressive disease, with no known cure, except that the course of the disease can be "arrested" if the patient commits to a lifelong goal of total abstinence. Clients who are reluctant to accept this premise are accused of being in total denial as to the true nature of their problem. Those who are unwilling to pursue abstinence-based treatment (ranging from pharmacotherapy to participation in 12-step groups) are often denied any treatment assistance. Therapists from this tradition often adopt a confrontational treatment approach designed to break down the patient's resistance to accepting the true biological nature of their illness. This approach is widely used, and includes a high incidence of therapeutic "interventions" in which the client is suddenly confronted by family and friends who have teamed up with a treatment program requiring immediate and total abstinence. Other confrontational treatment approaches include the use of "therapeutic communities" in which the client participates in an "encounter group" characterized by the use of direct and often negative feedback from other group members.

In contrast to the moral and disease models of addiction treatment, MBRP adopts the position that addiction has multiple causes and that it is a biopsychosocial problem, unique in its manifestation with each client. Just as there are several causes that determine the development of addictive problems, and that need to be explored with each client, there are also multiple pathways to resolution of the problem. This shift in underlying attitude is helpful if MBRP therapists are to facilitate a mindful attitude in their clientele, one characterized by nonjudgmental awareness and acceptance. It stands in sharp distinction to the moral model, with its emphasis on increasing self-blame, shame, guilt, and other aspects of stigma as the primary means of motivating change. The MBRP approach also differs strongly from the strict disease model, which focuses on breaking through denial, confronting clients, and convincing them that they are caught up in a progressive disease.

Although there are no official "therapists" in 12-step programs such as AA, clients are also told that they suffer from a chronic disease and must follow the 12 steps to recovery, with a reliance on belief in a "Higher Power" and participation in a spiritual self-help group. Clients are told that they each must follow the 12 steps in strict progression until they are firmly on the path to recovery. This path is the same for all, with little room for individual differences in the process of change. Total abstinence is the ultimate goal, and lifelong attendance at meetings is strongly advised. Recently, there has been some discussion about the parallel assumptions adopted by the 12-step community and the mindfulness-based approaches, given that both have been described as spiritual pathways to recovery (e.g., Griffin, 2004). Although the spiritual foundations are incorporated in both AA and MBRP approaches, MBRP therapists focus on *empowering* the client through personal practice, whereas AA encourages clients to give up their own power to some "Higher Power." In addition, MBRP therapists are more individual oriented in their approach to working with clients, and allow clients a choice of treatment goals other than total lifelong abstinence.

CONCLUSION

The quality of the therapeutic alliance in the treatment of addictive behavior problems is perhaps the most critical factor in determining treatment outcome. There is evidence in the literature that the nature of the alliance between therapist and client may carry more impact as a mediator of outcome than the theoretical orientation or intervention approach applied by the treatment provider. In an investigation comparing three different treatment modalities for alcohol dependence (cognitive-behavioral therapy, 12-step facilitation, and motivational interviewing), the research team conducting Project Match (Project MATCH Research Group, 1998) tried to investigate the role of various potential mediators of treatment outcome, including client personality factors, demographics, motivation for change, and drinking patterns. The only factor that was predictive of treatment success was the quality of the therapeutic alliance (determined by objective ratings of therapy sessions and the self-report evaluations made by both clients and therapists). Clients who had positive alliances with their therapists did better overall in terms of changes in drinking behavior, regardless of the specific therapeutic model being applied. This is an important finding and has strong implications for developing the positive therapeutic relationship that is fundamental to the successful implementation of MBRP.

Several empirical investigations of MBRP are currently under way, including randomized controlled trials assessing the effectiveness of MBRP in comparison to other empirically supported treatments. Because MBRP is still in its early stages of development, the protocol will continue to evolve and strengthen. The egalitarian, compassionate relationships between clients and therapists, however, are a core element in creating an environment that supports venturing into new territory and making fundamental changes in relating to and experiencing one's internal and external world. Respecting each individual's unique experience, goals, and readiness for change is fundamental to creating such an environment and will remain at the center of the MBRP stance and treatment protocol.

REFERENCES

Bender, E. (2007) Most substance-abusing inmates fail to get treatment. *Psychiatric News,* 42, 36.

Bowen, S., Witkiewitz, K., Dillworth, T. M., Chawla, N., Simpson, T. L., Ostafin, B., et al. (2006). Mindfulness meditation and substance use in an incarcerated population. *Psychology of Addictive Behaviors, 20,* 343–347.

Bowen, S., Witkiewitz, K., Dillworth, T. M., & Marlatt, G. A. (2007). The role of thought suppression in the relationship between mindfulness meditation and substance use. *Addictive Behaviors, 32*(10), 2324–2328.

Breslin, F. C., Zack M., & McMain, S. (2002). An information-processing analysis of mindfulness: Implications for relapse prevention in the treatment of substance abuse. *Clinical Psychology: Science and Practice, 9*(3), 275–299.

Brickman, P., Rabinowitz, V. C., Karuza, J., Coates, D., Cohn, E., & Kidder, L. (1982). Models of helping and coping. *American Psychologist, 37,* 368–384.

Carroll, K. M. (1996). Relapse prevention as a psychosocial treatment: A review of controlled clinical trials. *Experimental and Clinical Psychopharmacology, 4*(1), 46–54.

Cummings, C., Gordon, J. R., & Marlatt, G. A. (1980). Relapse: Strategies of prevention and prediction. In W. R. Miller (Ed.), *The addictive behaviors: Treatment of alcoholism, drug abuse, smoking, and obesity* (pp. 291–321). Oxford, UK: Pergamon Press.

Denning, P., Little, J., & Glickman, A. (2003). *Over the influence: The harm reduction guide for managing alcohol and drugs.* New York: Guilford Press.

Griffin, K. (2004). *One breath at a time: Buddhism and the twelve steps to recovery.* New York: Rodale.

Groves, P., & Farmer, R. (1994). Buddhism and addictions. *Addiction Research, 2,* 183–194.

Hart, W. (1987). *The art of living: Vipassana meditation as taught by S. N. Goenka.* San Francisco: HarperCollins.

Irvin, J. E., Bowers, C. A., Dunn, M. E., & Wang, M. C. (1999). Efficacy of relapse prevention: A meta-analytic review. *Journal of Consulting and Clinical Psychology, 67*(4), 563–570.

Jellinek, E. M. (1960). *The disease concept in alcoholism.* New Brunswick, NJ: Hill House Press.

Kabat-Zinn, J. (1982). An outpatient program in behavioral medicine for chronic pain patients based on the practice of mindfulness meditation: Theoretical considerations and preliminary results. *General Hospital Psychiatry, 4,* 33–42.

Kabat-Zinn, J. (1990). *Full catastrophe living.* New York: Delacorte.

Kadden, R. M. (2001). Behavioral and cognitive-behavioral treatment for alcoholism research opportunities. *Addictive Behaviors, 26,* 489–507.

Larimer, M., Palmer, R. S., & Marlatt, G. A. (1999). Relapse prevention: An overview of Marlatt's cognitive behavioral model. *Alcohol Research and Health, 23,* 151–169.

Marlatt, G. A. (1978). Craving for alcohol, loss of control, and relapse: A cognitive-behavioral analysis. In P. E. Nathan, G. A. Marlatt, & T. Loberg (Eds.), *Alcoholism: New directions in behavioral research and treatment* (pp. 271–314). New York: Plenum Press.

Marlatt, G. A. (1998). *Harm reduction: Pragmatic strategies for managing high-risk behaviors.* New York: Guilford Press.

Marlatt, G. A. (2002). Buddhist philosophy and the treatment of addictive behavior. *Cognitive and Behavioral Practice, 9,* 44–50.

Marlatt, G. A., & Donovan, D. M. (Eds.). (2005). *Relapse prevention: Maintenance strategies in the treatment of addictive behaviors* (2nd ed.). New York: Guilford Press.

Marlatt, G. A., & Gordon, J. R. (Eds.). (1985). *Relapse prevention: Maintenance strategies in the treatment of addictive behaviors.* New York: Guilford Press.

Marlatt, G. A., & Kristeller, J. (1999). Mindfulness and meditation. In W. R. Miller (Ed.), *Integrating spirituality in treatment: Resources for practitioners* (pp. 67–84). Washington, DC: APA Books.

Marlatt, G. A., Parks, G. A., Witkiewitz, K., Dillworth, T., Bowen, S., & Lonzcak, H. (2004). Mindfulness, addictive behaviors, and Vipassana meditation. In S. Hayes, M. Linehan,

& V. Follette (Eds.), *The new behavior therapies: Expanding the cognitive-behavioral tradition.* New York: Guilford Press.

Miller, W. R., & Rollnick, S. (2002). *Motivational interviewing: Preparing people for change* (2nd ed.). New York: Guilford Press.

Pelissier, B., Rhodes, W., Saylor, W., Gaes, G., Camp, S. D., Vanyur, S. D., et al. (2000). Triad drug treatment evaluation project: Final report of three-year outcomes: Part 1. *Federal Bureaus of Prisons Office of Research and Evaluation.*

Prochaska, J. O., & DiClemente, C. C. (1982). Transtheoretical therapy: Toward a more integrative model of change. *Psychotherapy: Theory, Research, and Practice, 19,* 276–288.

Project MATCH Research Group. (1998). Matching alcoholism treatments to client heterogeneity: Project MATCH three-year drinking outcomes. *Alcoholism: Clinical and Experimental Research, 22*(6), 1300–1311.

Rogers, C. R. (1959). A theory of therapy, personality, and interpersonal relationships, as developed in the client-centered framework. In S. Koch (Ed.), *Psychology: A study of a science* (Vol. 3). New York: McGraw-Hill.

Segal, Z., Teasdale, J. D., & Williams, M. (2002). *Mindfulness-based cognitive therapy for depression.* New York: Guilford Press.

Shiffman, S., Hickcox, M., Paty, J. A., Gnys, M., Kassel, J. D., & Richards, T. J. (1996). Progression from a smoking lapse to relapse: Prediction from abstinence violation effects, nicotine dependence, and lapse characteristics. *Journal of Consulting and Clinical Psychology, 64,* 993–1002.

Tatarsky, A. (2002). *Harm reduction psychotherapy: A new treatment for drug and alcohol problems.* Northvale, NJ: Jason Aronson.

Teasdale, J. D., Segal, Z., & Williams, J. M. G. (1995). How does cognitive therapy prevent depressive relapse and why should control (mindfulness) training help? *Behaviour Research and Therapy, 33,* 25–39.

Teasdale, J. D., Segal, Z. V., & Williams, J. M. G. (2003). Mindfulness training and problem formulation. *Clinical Psychology: Science and Practice, 10*(2), 157–160.

Witkiewitz, K., & Marlatt, G. A. (2004). Relapse prevention for alcohol and drug problems: That was Zen, this is Tao. *American Psychologist, 59*(4), 224–235.

Witkiewitz, K., & Marlatt, G. A. (2007). *Therapist's guide to evidence-based relapse prevention.* New York: Elsevier.

Witkiewitz, K., Marlatt, G. A., & Walker, D. D. (2005). Mindfulness-based relapse prevention for alcohol use disorders: The meditative tortoise wins the race. *Journal of Cognitive Psychotherapy, 19,* 221–228.

8 Mindfulness, Metacommunication, and Affect Regulation in Psychoanalytic Treatment

JEREMY D. SAFRAN
ROMY READING

Both Western psychotherapy and Buddhism share the goals of fostering transformation and alleviating suffering. These common goals have inspired a long-standing dialogue between the two traditions. In this chapter we focus specifically on the cross-fertilization that is beginning to take place between Buddhism and contemporary psychoanalytic practice. In the 1950s and 1960s some psychoanalysts were inspired by a flurry of interest in Buddhism, especially as seen in the works of Erich Fromm and Karen Horney. However, until recent years this interest had not had a significant impact on mainstream psychoanalysis. In the last decade, however, the dialogue between psychoanalysis and Buddhism has accelerated, resulting in an exchange of wisdom that has begun to transform both traditions (Epstein, 1995; Rubin, 1996; Safran, 2003, 2006). In this chapter we will focus specifically on the use of mindfulness practice as a tool for enhancing the therapist's ability to work constructively with the therapeutic relationship from a contemporary psychoanalytic perspective.

Mindfulness, as described in Buddhist technical treatises dating as far back as the third century B.C.E., can be conceptualized as the process of locating and directing one's awareness to the present moment as it unfolds. Essential to the development of this awareness is the simultaneous cultivation of self-acceptance and nonjudgment. The goal of mindfulness is to guide one to deautomate habitual ways of thinking, relating, and behaving. In what follows we examine a form of dialogical mindfulness practice, referred to as *therapeutic metacommunication*. We also provide background from theoretical developments in affect regulation. Therapeutic metacommunication is conceptualized as a form of *mindfulness in action* through which the therapist engages the patient in an ongoing collaborative exploration of patterns that unfold in the therapeutic relationship.

RELATIONAL PATTERNS AND ENACTMENTS

One of the most important changes that have taken place in the psychoanalytic tradition in the last two decades has been the shift from a view of the therapist as a neutral observer who stands outside of the relational field to a view in which the therapist is seen as an inextricable participant in the co-creation of the clinical situation. According to this paradigm shift, the therapist is an engaged participant whose subjectivity and emotional responsiveness interact with that of the patient, creating an interactional dynamic that constitutes the therapeutic relationship (Aron, 1996; Benjamin, 1988; Mitchell, 1988, 2000; Safran & Muran, 2000). Both the therapist and patient are understood to contribute consciously and unconsciously to the emergent therapeutic relationship. Everything that takes place in the therapy session is thus viewed as an ongoing co-creation of both participants in the therapeutic dyad. An ongoing exploration of this co-constructed reality and the interactional patterns of which it consists is considered essential to the therapeutic process.

All relational patterns that unfold in the therapeutic relationship can be understood as expressions of the patient's and therapist's unique personal histories, conflicts, and ways of relating to the world. In contemporary psychoanalytic theory, these relational patterns are conceptualized as involving unconscious contributions by both therapist and patient, and are termed *enactments* (e.g., Aron, 1996; Jacobs, 1991). An individual's generalized expectations about self–other interactions, known as *relational schemas*, shape his or her interpersonal perceptions. These relational schemas and perceptions guide, both consciously and unconsciously, the interpersonal strategies, actions, and interactions that unfold between the individual and other people. Each person's schemas can elicit varied reactions from the other, depending on the other's own unique relational schemas. For example, dominance may evoke submissiveness in one person and anger in another, while hostility may elicit compliance in one individual and further hostility in another. The interactional outcome is an emergent process that depends upon the conscious and unconscious contributions of both individuals in the moment.

In contemporary psychoanalytic thinking two assumptions can be made concerning these enactments. First, the therapist and patient themselves will inevitably become unconsciously *embedded* in enactments that reflect their unique characteristics. Second, the characteristic relational patterns that emerge between the patient and therapist may in some ways reflect patterns that emerge for the patient in his or her interpersonal relations outside of therapy. Although these enactments can obstruct the therapeutic process if they remain unexamined, they can also serve as fertile soil out of which constructive therapeutic process can grow. By working through therapeutic enactments in a mindful way, therapists and patients can discover internal processes and relational patterns that are problematic for patients and provide them with new, constructive relational experiences that modify their maladaptive relational schemas.

The process of disembedding from enactments involves an ongoing collaborative exploration between the therapist and the patient. To the extent that the therapist can collaborate in the process of becoming aware of and disembedding from the enactment, the patient will be able to engage in a new type of relational experience. Over time new relational experiences of this type can begin to modify maladaptive relational schemas or beliefs that shape the patient's interpersonal relationships outside of therapy. In addition, this process of collaboratively exploring enactments can help patients develop mindfulness skills that will be useful in deautomating their own unconscious self-defeating patterns in relationships with others. This is particularly important, since as noted earlier, there will be both similarities and differences between the therapeutic relationship and other relationships in the patient's life. The cultivation of relational mindfulness skills through the ongoing, collaborative exploration of the therapeutic relationship thus helps patients to cultivate a generalizable skill that they can use in their everyday lives.

MINDFULNESS AND DISEMBEDDING

When therapist and patient become embedded in an enactment, their contributions to the process exist outside of or on the fringes of awareness. The therapist's task is to engage the patient in a collaborative process of exploring these enactments in an attempt to discover how each of them is contributing. Through a type of mindful investigation, enactments can gradually be transformed into opportunities for awakening. For both patient and therapist, participation in an enactment is partially maintained by a disowning or dissociation of aspects of self-experience that are threatening or unacceptable. For example, the therapist who is embedded in a power struggle with his patient will have difficulty stepping outside of this struggle if he has difficulty acknowledging that he feels threatened or competitive. The therapist who is being critical or abusive toward her patients will have difficulty stepping outside of this enactment if she has difficulty acknowledging that she is feeling angry. It is for this reason that the skill of mindfulness becomes invaluable in facilitating the process of disembedding.

In the Buddhist tradition, the goal of mindfulness practice is to ultimately realize that all phenomena are inherently "empty" of any intrinsic, separate existence. In the psychoanalytic practice the emphasis is not on coming to experience the intrinsic emptiness of all phenomena but rather to become aware of dissociated feelings and actions and to use them as an important source of information. Two objectives can be articulated. First, mindfulness practice can enable the therapist to cultivate a sense of *internal space* by decreasing his or her attachment to any particular feeling. Within this opening of *internal space* new possibilities for potentially constructive therapeutic work emerge. We discuss this notion of internal space in greater detail later. Second, mindfulness allows therapists to refine their attentional skills so that awareness of their inner experience and their contributions to enactments can serve as an important source of information for the therapeutic process.

As stated previously mindfulness involves learning to locate and direct one's attention in an *accepting* and *nonjudgmental* fashion to one's thoughts, feelings, fantasies, and actions as they emerge in the present moment. Although it is recognized as inevitable that at times individuals who are attending to their experience mindfully will feel critical of their experience or themselves, the practice of mindfulness involves taking this judgment itself as the focus of awareness rather than tying to change it or avoid it. In this way the judgment itself begins to lose some of its potency. Through this process, a type of "letting go" or surrender begins to emerge for the therapist, and the experience of internal constriction associated with the need to dissociate experiences is replaced by an experience of internal space. Mindfulness enables therapists to cultivate a state of mind that allows them to work with their own internal experience so as to negotiate their way from a place devoid of possibilities for constructive therapeutic work to one in which acceptance and surrender allow for new possibilities to emerge (Safran & Muran, 2000; Safran 2003, 2006).

METACOMMUNICATION: MINDFULNESS IN ACTION

As previously indicated, a key tool for applying mindfulness practice to the collaborative exploration of enactments consists of therapeutic metacommunication—communicating about the implicit communication that is being enacted in the therapeutic relationship. The patient may, for example, be explicitly saying to the therapist: "Nobody is there for me" and implicitly saying, "You're not there for me." A therapist may explicitly be saying to the patient, "What's going on in our relationship is similar to what goes on for you in your relationships with other people" and implicitly be saying, "The problem is yours, not mine." Metacommunication is a type of mindfulness in action that involves investigating the nature and meaning of these implicit communications. A collaborative effort is made to bring an ongoing awareness to the interaction between the therapist and patient as it unfolds in the moment.

Essential to metacommunication is the therapist's ability to become as grounded as possible in her immediate experience of her own feelings or some aspect of the therapeutic relationship. Metacommunication requires that the therapist use her own feelings as a point of departure for the collaborative exploration. Various forms of metacommunication are possible. The therapist may, for example, provide the patient with feedback about the impact that the patient is having on her, for example, "I feel cautious with you . . . as if I am walking on eggshells." Or "I feel like it's difficult to really make contact with you. On the one hand, the things that you're talking about really seem important. But on the other, there is a subtle level at which it's difficult for me to really feel you." Or "I feel judged by you." All these expressions of feedback can serve to open up an exploration of the patient's inner experience. For example, the therapist can add, "Does this feedback make any sense to you? Do you have any awareness of judging me?" In some cases the patient will answer yes and further exploration can lead to a deeper understanding of his or her inner experience. In other cases, the patient will answer no. In such cases, it is possible that the therapist's feeling of being judged reflects her own contribution more than the patient's. Or alternatively, the patient may be judging the therapist but unable to become aware of this in the moment. As long as this feedback is offered in a tentative and exploratory fashion, however, no harm will be done, and when the time is ripe the therapist will be able to metacommunicate in a fashion that facilitates greater awareness in the patient. It can also be beneficial for the therapist to point directly to the specific instances of the patient's eliciting actions. "I feel dismissed or closed out by you, and I think that may be because you tend to not pause or reflect in way that would indicate that you are really considering what I am saying." All of these statements are intended to bring an ongoing awareness to the interaction as it unfolds in the moment. Below we outline some general principles of metacommunication. For a more detailed description the reader is referred to Safran and Muran (2000).

PRINCIPLES OF METACOMMUNICATION

1. *Explore with skillful tentativeness and emphasize one's own subjectivity.* The communication by the therapist should be exploratory. Rather than aiming to convey an objective tone, therapists should emphasize their own subjectivity. This approach is very much in accordance with the understanding in contemporary psychoanalytic thinking that the therapist's presence is not meant to be authoritative but instead collaborative. It is also vital to stress that the message at both the explicit and implicit levels should be one of inviting patients to engage in a collaborative attempt to understand what is taking place. Emphasizing the subjectivity of the therapist's perception encourages patients to use his or her observations as a stimulus for self-exploration rather than feeling compelled to react to either positive or negative authoritative statements.

2. *Do not assume a parallel with other relationships.* Although the process of metacommunication serves as a means for disembedding from enactments and, over time, modifies maladaptive relational schemas about self–other interactions, therapists should be concerned about prematurely attempting to establish a link between the configuration that is being enacted in the therapeutic relationship and other relationships in the patient's life. Although such parallels can be illuminating in some contexts, they can also be experienced by patients as blaming. In keeping with the principles of mindfulness, the focus should be on exploring the patients' internal experiences in a nuanced fashion, as they emerge in the moment.

3. *Ground all formulations in awareness of your own feelings and accept responsibility for your own contributions.* Therapists should always

begin by attempting to reflect on their own emergent emotions. Failure to do so may increase the level of distortion that stems from unconscious elements. Taking responsibility for one's own contributions to the interaction is vital. Since each participant is contributing to the interaction in ways of which they are unaware, it is essential to continually attempt to clarify the nature of the contribution. The process of explicitly acknowledging responsibility for one's contributions can be a potent intervention at times. First, the process can help patients to also become aware of unconscious or semiconscious feelings that they may have difficulty articulating. For example, acknowledging that one has been critical can help patients to articulate their feelings of hurt and resentment. Second, by validating the patient's perception of the therapist's actions, the therapist is able to reduce his or her own need for defensiveness.

4. *Start where you are.* The ability to remain anchored in the moment, which is central to mindfulness practice, will greatly serve the process of metacommunication. Collaborative exploration of the therapeutic relationship should take into account the feelings, intuitions, and observations that are emerging for the therapist and patient in the moment. It is critical to understand that what was true in one session may not be true in the next and what was true in one moment may change in the next moment. For example, while a therapist may be able to adopt an empathic response toward an aggressive patient in one moment, another moment may lead the therapist to a space in which she cannot feel empathic. Instead, the therapist must begin by first fully accepting and working with her own feelings and subjective reactions to the patient's expression of aggression as it occurs in the moment. From there further collaborative understanding can follow.

5. *Evaluate and explore patients' responses to interventions.* Patients' responsiveness to interventions must continuously be monitored and explored. It is important to understand if patients are using the therapist's intervention as a stimulus for further investigation or if they are responding in a way that is inhibiting further understanding. Do they respond in a minimal fashion without elaboration? Do they not respond at all? Do they respond in a defensive or self-justifying fashion? Do they agree too readily in what appears to be an attempt to be a "good" patient? It is essential that therapists mindfully attend to their own subtle intuitions about the quality of a patient's responsiveness, and carefully acknowledge any sensation linked to a patient's response. For example, the therapist may feel at some level that the patient has an ambivalent response to an intervention, even though the therapist may have diffi-

culty articulating what cues these feelings are based on. If and when an intervention fails to deepen exploration or in fact further inhibits such exploration, it is vital that the therapist explore the way in which the patient has experienced the intervention. Did the patient experience the therapist's intervention as critical, blaming, or accusatory? Did he or she experience it as domineering, demanding, or manipulative? Over time, this type of collaborative exploration can help to articulate the nature of the enactments that are taking place. In addition, these very explorations can serve to guide patients toward understanding their characteristic ways of construing interpersonal relationships and gradually lead to a fleshing out of their unique relational schemas.

6. *Collaborative exploration of the therapeutic relationship and disembedding take place at the same time.* A clear formulation of what is occurring in the context of the enactment is not a necessary prerequisite to initiating the metacommunication process. In fact the very process of articulating one's own perceptions and feelings as they arise in the moment can lead to a more authentic formulation that will be grounded in a collaboration with the patient. Moreover, the process of telling patients about an aspect of one's experience that one is in conflict over can open the internal space so that the therapist is free to see the situation with more clarity. For example, a therapist who is feeling resentful toward a patient who does not respect his boundaries judges himself harshly for feeling resentful, dissociates his negative feelings, and experiences a collapse of internal space that prevents him from responding creatively to the situation. In this situation, it might be helpful for the therapist to say something like "I feel anxious about saying this because I'm afraid of hurting your feelings, but I think I've been feeling a bit irritated because it feels like my boundaries are being pushed against." The process of putting what feels unsayable into words begins to reopen the therapist's internal space.

7. *Remember that an attempt to explore what is taking place in the therapeutic relationship can function as a new cycle of an ongoing unconscious enactment.* Any metacommunication can itself be an enactment. For example, the therapist may articulate a growing intuition that the patient is withdrawing, and say, "It feels to me like I'm trying to pull teeth." Perhaps as a result of perceiving the therapist's unconscious defensive contribution, the patient withdraws even further and the interpersonal dance intensifies, with the therapist escalating his attempts to break through and the patient only becoming more defended. Therefore it is critical to track the quality of patient responsiveness to all interventions and especially to examine their experience of interventions that

have not been facilitative. The therapist must ask, does the intervention deepen the patient's self-exploration or lead to defensiveness or compliance? The process of exploring the way in which patients experience interventions that are not facilitative helps to refine the understanding of the unconscious interpersonal dance that is taking place in the moment.

THE THERAPIST'S MIND AS AN INSTRUMENT OF CHANGE

When metacommunication enables the therapist and patient to disembed from an enactment, it does so not just because the therapist has found the right words, but also because the words reflect the fact that the therapist has managed to enter into the right state of mind. Metacommunication not only helps patients to become aware of their relational patterns, it helps the therapist enter into a therapeutic state of mind by putting into words that which feels unspeakable (Safran & Muran, 2000). To speak about the therapist's *state of mind*, however, does not do justice to the nondual nature of the mind–body relationship. A more accurate phrase would be the therapist's *embodied state of being*. The mind is embodied and the patient–therapist interaction, like all other human interactions, involves a process of mutual influence and regulation at a bodily felt level. The heart of the therapeutic process involves affective communication at both conscious and unconscious levels (Safran & Muran, 2000).

In order to understand the significance of this point it is worth taking a brief detour into the realm of emotion theory and research. There is a movement afoot in diverse therapeutic traditions to develop a comprehensive motivational theory grounded in contemporary emotion theory and research (e.g., Greenberg & Safran, 1987; Jones, 1995; Lichtenberg, 1989; Safran & Greenberg, 1991; Spezzano, 1993). Central to this theory is the notion that emotions are biologically wired into the human organism through an evolutionary process and that they play an adaptive role in the survival of the species. Emotions function to safeguard the concerns of the organism (Ekman & Davidson, 1994; Frijda, 1986; Spezzano, 1993). Some of these concerns or goals are biologically programmed (e.g., attachment), while others are learned. Emotions are conceptualized as a form of action disposition information. They provide us with internal feedback about the actions that we are prepared to engage in, as well as information about the self as a biological organism with a particular history in interaction with the environment. As such, they are at the core of subjective and intersubjective meaning.

It is useful to understand the structure underlying the fundamental sequences of social behavior in terms of motivational systems that have been wired into the human species through a process of natural selection. Examples include attachment, exploration, sexual excitement, flight, and aggression (e.g., Bowlby, 1988; Jones, 1995; Spezzano, 1993). Emotions function as the subjective readout (or experiential monitor) of which motivational systems or combinations of them are dominant at any given time. These systems become activated in response to the appraisal (which is typically only partially conscious) of various environmental contingencies. For example, anger occurs in response to events experienced as an assault or violation. It informs the individual of his or her organismic preparedness to engage in self-protective behavior. Sadness occurs in response to a loss and organismically prepares one to recover or compensate for what is lost. Fear is evoked by events appraised as dangerous and informs individuals of an organismic preparedness for flight. Emotions can thus be thought of as a type of *embodied knowledge.*

While emotion provides the individual with a monitor of his or her own action dispositions, the expressive-motor behaviors associated with it provide others with an ongoing readout of these same action dispositions. While this process of reading the other's affective displays can have a conscious element to it, a good deal of it takes place out of awareness, in the same way that other affective appraisals take place. Thus, for example, we may unconsciously appraise the other's aggressive disposition toward us, and in turn feel angry (i.e., be prepared to reciprocate with aggression), without being fully aware of either our own readiness to be aggressive or the cues to which we are responding. Moreover, we may be unconsciously responding to an action disposition that the other may be unaware of. As Parkinson (1995) suggests in his review of the literature on affective communication, "Moment-by moment reactions to another person's displays are not mediated by any conscious emotional conclusions about what these expressions signify, but rather are part of one's skilled and automatized engagement in interpersonal life, and one's ecological attunement to the unfolding dynamic aspects of the situation" (p. 279).

Healthy functioning thereby involves the integration of affective information with higher-level cognitive processing in order to act in a fashion that is grounded in organismically based need, but not bound by reflexive action (Greenberg & Safran, 1987; Leventhal, 1984; Safran & Greenberg, 1991). Thus, for example, an individual may be aware of his anger at someone but deem it unwise to respond aggressively. Individuals who have difficulty accessing the full range of their emotional experience, however, will be deprived of important information. They may suppress or fail to mobilize a motivational system that may be adaptive in a specific context. For example, the individual who has difficulty experiencing anger may fail to mobilize adaptive aggression. The individual who has difficulty experiencing more vulnerable feelings may fail to fulfill healthy needs for nurturance. A second consequence of the process of dissociating emotional experience is that there may be incongruence between one's actions and subjective experience. Since the activation of a motivational system is not dependent on the conscious experience of the associated emotion, it is not uncommon for people to have only partial awareness of the impact they have on others. Thus, for example, the individual who dissociates feelings of anger may nevertheless act aggressively and evoke aggression in response. This type of incongruent communication can play a major role in psychopathology and in the type of therapeutic enactments discussed previously.

There is growing evidence that a range of psychopathologies involve deficits in the capacity for affect regulation (Schore, 2003). Affect regulation involves tolerating, modulating, and making constructive use of a range of different affective states, including those that are intensely painful or pleasurable, without needing to dissociate them. People initially develop the capacity for affect regulation through their interactions with their attachment figures. As infant researchers have shown, there is an ongoing process of mutual affective regulation between mothers and infants through which both partners influence each other's affective states (Beebe & Lachmann, 2002; Tronick, 1989). In a healthy developmental process there is an optimal balance between interactive regulation and self-regulation. There are periods when the mother and infant are affectively coordinated with one another and periods when they are not. When this process becomes derailed there is an excess of one of the two types of affect regulation (i.e., either an excess of interactive regulation or an excess of self-regulation). Thus for example, the mother who is excessively dependent on emotional contact with her infant will pursue eye contact with him in an attempt to elicit a smile even after he has averted his gaze. Or alternatively, the child who learns that parents respond to her own painful feelings (e.g., anxiety, anger) with catastrophic responses of their own (e.g., panicking or becoming excessively angry) will learn to attempt to regulate her feelings on her own. Without having the experience of learning that these feelings are tolerable within the relationship, however, he or she will never develop the capacity to self-regulate in a healthy fashion and will not be able to learn to use relationships in a healthy fashion to help regulate painful or distressing feelings.

In treatment, therapists' ability to resonate with their patients' more painful emotions and to tolerate the intensely painful and frightening emotions that can be evoked in them during enactments can be transformative for patients in and of itself. This type of containment (to use the psychoanalyst Wilfred Bion's term), in which therapists process emotions evoked in them by patients in a nondefensive way, can be a powerful way of helping them to learn that relationships will not necessarily be destroyed by painful, aggressive, or potentially divisive feelings and that they themselves can survive these feelings. To be able to provide this type of affect regulation or containment for the patient, however, therapists require the capacity to regulate their own difficult or painful feelings in a constructive fashion. Psychoanalysts have always maintained that the therapist's capacity to manage difficult feelings evoked in him or her during the treatment (what are referred to as countertransference feelings) is a critical therapeutic skill. It has been assumed that one develops this capacity through undergoing one's own personal treatment. And to the extent that the capacity for affect regulation develops as a result of healthy developmental experiences (and therapy is conceptualized in part as a healthy developmental experience), this seems reasonable. The cultivation of an ongoing mindfulness practice in combination with the practice of therapeutic metacommunication can, however, play a valuable role in helping therapists to further refine this capacity.

A CLINICAL ILLUSTRATION

We now examine a brief clinical illustration of the process of metacommunication. Since our emphasis here is on clinical process rather than case conceptualization no information is provided about the background or details of the case. The transcript is taken from an early session with a desperate and angrily demanding patient whom we call Silvia.[1]

THERAPIST: So this is our second session together, and I am wondering what you're feeling, and whether you have any thoughts or questions after our last session.

SILVIA: I'm not very happy. I'm very frustrated with you, actually. Last time, I came in here, just sat here, and I talked and talked and talked. And nothing, absolutely nothing. You sat there, the way you are sitting there now, and you didn't really say much of anything, and I—it's angering me because if I'm supposed to come—if I'm going to therapy, if I'm going here and I'm doing this, I want an answer. I can't just talk and talk and talk and have you say things that lead me in an abstract way. How is this gonna work? I need to know from you how is this going to work? I need a concrete answer. How do I get from where I am now to somewhere else? I need a way to go. I . . . don't know how to go. I've been in therapy for 2 years and nothing seems to be helping. And you're not helping either. So, it's like, what do I do?

THERAPIST: OK, so you know, I'm hearing that you're not happy about our last session and that you're feeling frustrated and also, if I understand correctly, that you'd like to hear more from me as to what—about how the therapy works . . .

SILVIA: How do you do work? How do you do what you do? How is this supposed to help me? How do I fix what's going on?

THERAPIST: OK, I'll try to answer that. . . . But before I say anything, I want to say that I have some concern about whether or not whatever I'm going to say is what you're really wanting. But I'll do my best, OK. . . . you have a funny look on your face. . . .

SILVIA: I'm not sure why you're concerned about that. Isn't that your job? To tell me how things are supposed to go . . . I'm confused then.

Silvia begins the session by expressing her anger and frustration with the way things have been going and by pressuring the therapist to provide her with an explanation of how therapy is going to help her. The therapist metacommunicates his concern that it is going to be difficult to satisfy her and then, picking up on her exasperated look, begins to explore her reaction to his metacommunication. Although this first attempt at metacommunication has not yet led to a positive shift in the quality of the therapeutic relationship, it has initiated the process of helping the therapist to enter into a more therapeutic state of mind. By attending to his experience rather than responding to the pressure and discomfort he feels without awareness, and by putting his intuitions into words, he begins to regulate his own affect and is able to avoid responding in an overly defensive way.

THERAPIST: Yeah, I mean it is my job to do my best to help you and to try and answer your questions, yeah, but there is something about . . . it's a bit difficult for me to put into words . . . but something about the intensity with which you are asking for things which makes me a little bit . . . which leads me to question my ability to give you the answer that you're wanting. But I'll try . . . OK? Basically as I see it, the way in which therapy works is that the two of us will work together to explore things that you may not be completely aware of . . . ways that you may see things that are self-defeating or ways in which you are dealing with your feelings that are self-defeating, or ways in which . . . you're shaking your head.

SILVIA: . . . I'm not defeating myself. I don't defeat myself. I don't understand how coming in here and working on it together is gonna help. Aren't I—isn't it supposed to be that I say what's going on and you tell me an answer—give me an answer? Isn't that the way it usually works? You ask a question, you get an answer. I don't understand what you're trying to do that would help. I don't think I'm defeating myself.

THERAPIST: Um-hmm.

SILVIA: I don't think I'm defeating myself at all.

THERAPIST: Um-hmm.

SILVIA: I think I come in here for answers and you're not giving them to me.

THERAPIST: Um-hmm. I'll certainly give you answers to the extent that I have them. But also some of it will have to come out of the two of us really exploring things together.

SILVIA: Yeah, that's too abstract for me. I need something concrete. I need to know how to get from point A to point B.

THERAPIST: Um-hmm.

SILVIA: And if I'm just gonna sit here and get this abstract stuff . . . it's kind of wasting my time, isn't it? It's kind of a waste of my time. That's what the past 2 years have been with other people. It's just a waste of my time if I just sit and get things in the abstract.

THERAPIST: Um-hmm, yeah, you know I'm trying to think if there is any way that I can be more concrete than I am right now. Um, let me . . . let me give you an example, OK?

SILVIA: OK, that's concrete.

THERAPIST: Even right now, let's try to take a look at what's going on between the two of us. You obviously, you want an answer, and I understand that you want an answer, and I want to give you what you
need. But I think there is something about the—just try to understand what's going on for me—there's something about the intensity
with which you're asking . . . the pressure where I'm supposed to
produce something, that makes it difficult for me to . . .

SILVIA: Isn't it your job? To produce something . . . to give me an answer? Isn't that your job?

THERAPIST: Well my job is to help you. But there's something about
what's going on between the two of us right now that's making it
difficult for me to really give you what you're wanting or needing.

SILVIA: Aren't you asking me to perform too? Aren't you asking me to
give you stuff too?

THERAPIST: Tell me more about that. Does it seem . . . ?

SILVIA: Aren't you asking me to tell you what's going on with me and articulate what's going on with me? So I'm being asked to perform
too? Aren't I?

THERAPIST: I'm wondering if you felt criticized by what I said just now.

SILVIA: Of course I did. I felt like you're blaming me. Like I came in here
and I was trying to say how I felt, and trying to say what I wanted
from you . . . and needed from you and it comes right back at me.

THERAPIST: OK . . . I need to think about that a little bit. I don't think it
was my intention to blame you . . . but maybe there was a way in
which I was responding out of feeling pressured, and maybe feeling
. . . feeling a little bit blamed for not giving you what you want. So
that in turn I was kind of blaming you. So it's kind of like passing a
hot potato back and forth. You know . . . like you're saying I'm not
doing my job, and I'm saying you're not doing your job. Does that
make any sense to you?

SILVIA: Yeah, a little, yeah.

THERAPIST: OK . . . so if that is what's going on between the two of us
. . . then . . . I'm not exactly sure how we're going to get past this . . .
but I think the two of us being able to agree that that is what's going
on is a start . . . right? And, I'm willing to work with you in order to
help the two of us find a way to get past this point. Right? And my
sense is that would be an important first step for us. OK?

SILVIA: OK, yeah, OK.

THERAPIST: OK.

Although the therapist suspects that any attempt to provide an answer to her question will fail, he attempts to provide a short formulation, on the assumption that not to do so will be experienced as an aggressive act and will exacerbate the situation even further. As expected, Silvia does not find the answer helpful, and she continues to express her anger and frustration. The therapist attempts to metacommunicate again by putting into words the way in which the pressure he feels from her makes it even more difficult for him to offer an answer that will feel helpful to her. Once again, this metacommunication is not immediately helpful to Silvia, but it continues to help the therapist attend to his experience in a mindful fashion and to regulate his own emotions.

This in turn makes it easier for the therapist to be open to further understanding Silvia's experience and reduces the possibility that he will exacerbate Silvia's affective disregulation through his own disregulated affect. When Silvia indicates that she feels pressured to perform as well, the therapist suspects that she has experienced his metacommunication as an accusation. Monitoring and exploring the patient's experience of the therapist's intervention is a key principle of metacommunication. In response to the therapist's probe, Silvia is able to acknowledge feeling blamed. The enactment begins to shift and the process of disembedding is under way. The therapist articulates what his motivations are and is able to acknowledge that perhaps he has been responding defensively to a feeling of being attacked. He frames things in terms of the vicious cycle that they are both caught in: "You're saying I am not doing my job, and I'm saying you're not doing your job." At this point Silvia begins to soften. Therapist and patient are beginning to shift to a more positive cycle of mutual affective regulation. The beginning of an alliance is established around the goal of collaborating to find their way out of this enactment.

Above and beyond any conceptual understanding that might emerge out of this interaction, the ability of Silvia and her therapist to begin the process of negotiating a more mutually responsive relationship at a bodily felt level is an important part of the work. Such processes as the therapist's ability to serve as a container for Silvia's anger and underlying feelings of helplessness and despair by tolerating his own negative feelings in a nondefensive way will ultimately help Silvia to experience her own negative feelings as more tolerable. By explicitly taking responsibility for his own negative feelings, the therapist begins the process of detoxifying the cycle of blame and counterblame and helps Silvia begin to tolerate and acknowledge her own feelings of anger and resentment. She thus has less of a need to see the hostility as originating exclusively from the therapist.

If this process continues over the course of treatment, Silvia will become less likely to experience the therapist as persecuting or depriving, and better able to acknowledge underlying feelings of despair, and eventually feelings of vulnerability and need as well. These more vulnerable underlying feelings are then able to actualize their adaptive potential by eliciting comfort and nurturance from the other. This in turn will make it easier for the therapist to genuinely empathize with Silvia and to provide the support and nurturance she so desperately needs. In this fashion a process of positive mutual affective regulation takes over time in which the therapist is able to help regulate Silvia's feelings by regulating his own feelings. As Silvia internalizes this constructive relational experience, she begins to develop new type of implicit relational knowing (Lyons-Ruth, 1998) that allows her to become better at using the other to help her regulate her affective experience and better at regulating her own affective experience as well.

CONCLUSION

There is a growing recognition in diverse therapeutic traditions that the relational and nonverbal aspects of the therapeutic process are as important as the verbal aspects. This is particularly true within contemporary psychoanalytic thinking. Building upon insights emerging from mother–infant developmental research, we have proposed a model of change in which the process of mutual affective regulation between therapist and patient lies at the core of the change process. Emotional dysregulation plays an important role in many forms of psychopathology, and the therapist's capacity to regulate his or her own emotions during therapeutic enactments and difficult therapeutic moments can be critical in the process of helping patients to learn to regulate their emotions more constructively, both through the use of the other and through self-regulation skills that emerge out of the process of mutual regulations between therapist and patient.

Mindfulness meditation provides a tool that therapists can use to help them develop a greater capacity to regulate their own affect so that they are better able to serve as surrogate affect regulators for their patients during therapeutic enactments. The internal skills acquired through mindfulness practice can also help therapists develop the skills to metacommunicate with their patients during enactments in order to help them both disembed from destructive relational scenarios, thereby providing patients with new relational experiences that will modify their internal models of self–other relationships. This process leads to a change in the patient's implicit relational knowing (Lyons-Ruth, 1998) about self–other relationships.

NOTE

1. This material is excerpted from Safran and Muran (2006). Copyright 2006 by Jeremy D. Safran. Reprinted by permission.

REFERENCES

Aron, L. (1996). *A meeting of minds: Mutuality in psychoanalysis.* Hillsdale, NJ: Analytic Press.

Beebe, B., & Lachmann, F. M. (2002). *Infant research and adult treatment.* Hillsdale, NJ: Analytic Press.

Benjamin, J. (1988). *The bonds of love.* New York: Pantheon Books.

Bowlby, J. (1988). *A secure base.* New York: Basic Books.

Ekman, P., & Davidson, R. J. (1994). *The nature of emotions: Fundamental questions.* New York: Oxford University Press.

Epstein, M. (1995). *Thoughts without a thinker.* New York: Basic Books.

Frijda, N. H. (1986). *The emotions.* New York: Cambridge University Press.

Greenberg, L. S., & Safran, J. D. (1987). *Emotion in psychotherapy.* New York: Guilford Press.

Jacobs, T. (1991). *The use of the self: Countertransference and communication in the analytic setting.* Madison, CT: International Universities Press.

Jones, J. M. (1995). *Affects as process: An inquiry into the centrality of affect in psychological life.* Hillsdale, NJ: Analytic Press.

Leventhal, H. (1984). A perceptual–motor theory of emotion. In L. Berkowitz (Ed.), *Advances in experimental social psychology* (pp. 117–182). New York: Academic Press.

Lichtenberg, J. (1989). *Psychoanalysis and motivation.* Hillsdale, NJ: Analytic Press.

Lyons-Ruth, K. (1998). Implicit relational knowing: Its role in development and psychoanalytic treatment. *Infant Mental Health Journal, 19,* 282–291.

Mitchell, S. A. (1988). *Relational concepts in psychoanalysis.* Cambridge, MA: Harvard University Press.

Mitchell, S. (2000). *Relationality: From attachment to intersubjectivity.* Hillsdale, NJ: Analytic Press.

Parkinson, B. (1995). *Ideas and realities of emotion.* London: Routledge.

Rubin, J. (1996). *Psychotherapy and Buddhism.* New York: Plenum Press.

Safran, J. D. (2003). Psychoanalysis and Buddhism as cultural institutions. In J. D. Safran

(Ed.), *Psychoanalysis and Buddhism: An unfolding dialogue* (pp. 1–34). Boston: Wisdom.

Safran, J. D. (2006). Before the ass has gone the horse has already arrived. *Contemporary Psychoanalysis, 42*, 197–212.

Safran, J. D., & Greenberg, L. S. (1991). *Emotion, psychotherapy, and change.* New York: Guilford Press.

Safran, J. D., & Muran, J. C. (2000). *Negotiating the therapeutic alliance: A relational treatment guide.* New York: Guilford Press.

Safran, J. D., & Muran, J. C. (2006). *Resolving therapeutic impasses* [DVD]. Santa Cruz, CA: Customflix.

Schore, A. N. (2003). *Affect dysregulation and disorders of the self.* New York: Norton.

Spezzano, C. (1993). *Affect in psychoanalysis.* Hillsdale, NJ: Analytic Press.

Tronick, E. (1989). Emotion and emotional communications in infants. *American Psychologist, 44*, 112–119.

9 Relational Mindfulness and Dialogic Space in Family Therapy

MISHKA LYSACK

As I looked at the picture, I could see dark storm clouds, rain, and lightning framing the edges, with several objects floating, suspended under the dark clouds in a sea of agitation. A boy of 10, accompanied by his mother (details changed to protect client privacy), was showing me his drawing about how "worry" overshadowed his life. The picture was devoid of human presence, except for two large hands stretching up from the bottom, straining, yearning for help but achingly empty. As the boy talked about his drawing, his agitation was almost palpable in the air, with his mother slumped in her chair, defeated, overcome with discouragement.

Amidst the voices of agitation and discouragement, I sensed other "voices" present in our conversation on the periphery of my awareness. As I focused on my breath and sank more deeply into the present moment, I began to notice echoes and resonances of more hopeful and peaceful voices (Bakhtin, 1984) that were absent, yet implicit in the conversational stream. I began to ask questions about these alternate voices in the flow of discussion; the boy sat back in his chair attentively as his mother began to sit up. After I described mindfulness to them as a way of decentering oneself from one's thoughts and outlined the practices that nurture this way of positioning oneself in the world, the boy was eager to "give it a try." After they had meditated together for a short time, the mother commented that this was similar to what they had learned in their first yoga class last week. Smiling, *amused by this synchronicity, I asked the boy to draw another picture for our next meeting, encouraging him and his mother to use the Kabat-Zinn CD in their mindfulness practices.*

Two weeks later, I found myself irresistibly drawn into the boy's excitement as he pointed to his picture. Instead of storm clouds and lightning, a yellow sun bathed the scene, birds and clouds drifting in the sky. The boy was now visible in the center of the picture, smiling and gesturing with his hand, surrounded by a number of "thought clouds" inscribed with several short phrases: "breath," "it's just a thought," "just forget about it," "it can't happen," "talk," and "be careful." Beside him, a purple-blue stream flowed off into the distant horizon, with the words "Let the thoughts float away" inscribed in the stream. Assuring me that they had practiced sitting meditation and the body scan since our last session, the boy and his mother described the differences that they had noticed in the relationship between "worry" and the boy. While worry was still present, they insisted that it was less influential, a series of "thought clouds" from which the boy was increasingly able to decenter himself as they floated in and out of his awareness.

MINDFULNESS AND DIALOGUE

In *Coming to Our Senses*, Jon Kabat-Zinn (2005) proposes a suggestive parallel between the qualities of individual mindfulness and attentive dialogue between persons. He suggests that "we speak of *dialogue* as the outer counterpart to the inward cultivation of moment-to-moment nonjudgmental awareness, or mindfulness" (p. 448). In his description of dialogue as an exterior form of mindfulness, Kabat-Zinn uses the metaphor of "voice" as a way of naming the events that arise within the field of awareness.

> Just as in the practice of mindfulness, we attend to whatever "voices" are arising in the mindspace and in the nowspace, hearing, feeling, touching, tasting, knowing the full spectrum of each arising, its lingering, its passing away, . . . so we can give ourselves over in the same way to being in conversation with others in dialogue. (p. 448)

In his exploration of the contours of this "space" between persons that is enacted through dialogue, Kabat-Zinn (2005) proposes that the attentive, nonjudgmental quality of the positioning of a person in mindfulness practices is also a characteristic of the interpersonal space in authentic dialogue. "Just as we need to feel open and safe in our own meditation practice, so we need to create enough openness and safety and spaciousness of heart for people in a meeting to feel safe in speaking their minds and from their hearts without having to worry about being judged by others" (p. 448). Kabat-Zinn highlights that dialogue, derived from the word *dialektos* (*dia* = between, *lectos* = to speak), designates a qualitatively different mode of interaction between persons, where the "quality of the relational space is the key to emergences and openings" (p. 450).

In proposing this parallel between *mindfulness* as the positioning of an individual in relation to the world and *dialogue* as attentive positioning of a person in relationship with others, I suggest that Kabat-Zinn offers us an important contribution to perceiving mindfulness and dialogue as comparable modes of action and being. While it is true that therapy consists of more than relational positioning and also includes the contributions and perspectives of the therapist, nonetheless, therapy may be conceptualized as a specialized mode of relating, characterized in part by a posture constituted by attentive listening and responsive dialogic interaction between client and therapist.

As a profession, family therapy focuses its attention on the relational spaces and the patterns of connection *between* persons in networks of relationships, advocating that the qualities of the therapeutic relationship contribute to the emergence of healing patterns in therapy. This relational positioning of oneself in an attentive posture of interaction is associated with particular micropractices of relationship and forms of moment-by-moment responsivity, facilitating healing processes in family relationships.

Within family therapy, there is a loosely affiliated cluster of theories and practices—which I would term "dialogic" approaches—that are influenced by social constructionism and center on the metaphors of "voice" and "dialogue" as a thematic thread in their understanding of clinical work. As a theoretical tradition, social constructionism "allows for a multiplicity of perspectives and a methodology of discourse that fosters multiple descriptions and alternative explanations of human experience. It offers a dialogic means to mediate contradictions and to co-construct solutions" (Tomm, 1998b, p. 173). Rather than seeing the relationship as a mere backdrop for therapeutic activity, these dialogic approaches to family therapy have devoted attention to the particular practices through which therapists may position themselves in responsive relationships with clients in order to foster the emergence of transformative *dialogue* as the context for the healing of relationships. Indeed, dialogic approaches in family therapy may be considered a form of co-meditation practice where intersubjectivity may be deepened through mindful listening to a form of "interbeing" and a compassionate witnessing of the suffering of others (Gehart & McCollum, 2007).

MEDITATION PRACTICES IN FAMILY THERAPY

Previous authors have explored the ways in which meditation may be integrated within individual or family therapy (Griffith & Griffith, 2002, pp. 182–185; Becvar, 2003; Simon, 1999; Wylie & Simon, 2004; Germer, Siegel, & Fulton, 2005). Meditation practices have been directed toward assisting clients to increase their sense of clarity, focused concentration, and mental stillness as well as to diminish physical suffering, tension, and pain (Bell, 1998) or to prevent depression relapse (Segal, Williams, & Teasdale, 2002). Germer (2005) provides an overview as to how practitioners may teach mindfulness to clients in therapy, outlining a comprehensive inventory of exercises and practices. Walsh (1999) has cautioned therapists working in the area of trauma "to proceed slowly and to prepare clients for whom difficult or painful memories and feelings may emerge, such as survivors of trauma, helping them to hold such experiences in a safe, bounded, and centered way that fosters their transformation" (p. 44). In many of these discussions, including the recent cognitive mindfulness and acceptance approaches (Hayes, Follette, & Linehan, 2004), little consideration has been given to the meditative practices of therapists and their role in the therapeutic relationship.

Some therapists (Schwartz, 1999; Simon, 1996) have suggested that psychotherapy itself could be reconceptualized as a spiritual practice for both the client and practitioner, but have focused their attention on the client, without any detailed discussion of the therapists themselves developing a meditative practice. Simon (1999) specifically advocated that therapists develop their own meditative practice as a way of cultivating mindfulness in their therapeutic presence with families, and as a way of strengthening the relationship rapport between the therapist and family members. Such authors have suggested that the meditative practice of a therapist can foster greater openness, responsiveness, and attentiveness on the part of the therapist, contributing to the practitioner's ability to remain focused when working with a family in which there are high levels of emotional distress and conflictual turmoil. For instance, Rosenthal (1990) proposes that meditative practices may also contribute to the effectiveness of clinical work by helping practitioners "avoid locking into preconceptions and fixed ideas that can close off the new possibilities arising in the therapeutic encounter" (pp. 40–41).

From my perspective, it is Segal and colleagues (2002) who provide the most engaging discussion of their movement from seeing mindfulness as merely a technique used by clients to gradually recognizing how they as therapists needed to develop their own mindfulness practices (pp. 43–63). In academic psychology, their account of their reorientation from traditional cognitive therapy to a mindfulness-based approach is refreshingly transparent. In a conversation with Kabat-Zinn, they provide a window into their initial misgivings about developing their own meditative practices, describing their subsequent journey into new territories for psychotherapy as they allowed the mindfulness-based stress reduction (MBSR) approach to transform their therapeutic model. Kabat-Zinn (2005, pp. 431–444) provides an intriguing alternate perspective on these generative conversations regarding the importance of therapists cultivating their own mindfulness practices.

In the area of practitioner education, Twemlow (2001a) has advocated mindfulness practices as part of the education of novice practitioners in core therapeutic principles as well as particular clinical practices, having developed links between Zazen meditation in Buddhism and individual psychoanalysis. More recently, Fulton (2005) and Morgan and Morgan (2005) have explored the relationship of mindfulness to clinical training for mental health professionals, and how mindfulness practices may contribute to the emergence of attention and empathy on the part of psychotherapists.

ENHANCING RELATIONAL MINDFULNESS IN FAMILY THERAPY

Theoretical Resources

Relational Stance in the Therapeutic Relationship

In their inquiry into the therapeutic relationship, family therapists have considered the relationship not as a static entity within which the family is merely an object to be passively observed, but rather as an ongoing active co-construction on the part of both the therapist and family. The relational stance taken by family therapists relative to the family has been variously termed an "emotional posture" (Griffith & Griffith, 1994), a "philosophical stance" (Anderson, 1997), an "ethical posture" (Tomm, 1998a), and a "relational and ethical stance for responsive practices" (Lysack, 2005). Writers have referred to the project of evoking the relational space that emerges between the therapist and the family as creating a "conversational domain" (Griffith & Griffith, 1994), a "dialogic space" for moving from monologue to dialogue (Penn & Frankfurt, 1994; Lysack, 2002; Pare & Lysack, 2004), "reflecting processes for inner and outer talk" (Andersen, 1992, 1995; Lysack, 2003), or a realm for the purpose of "co-constructing responsibility" (Tomm, 1998a).

For family therapists, making therapeutic distinctions "implies more than just passively observing an entity or phenomenon . . . It also entails actively adopting a certain position, a behavioral stance, or a 'posture' in relation to the entity or phenomenon distinguished" (Tomm, 1992, p. 119). This is somewhat similar to the *decentered* yet *affectionately attentive* posture that Kabat-Zinn (2005) describes as the mindfully oriented relationship between individuals and the events that arise in their own personal awareness. For family therapists, assuming such a relational stance in therapy also highlights the *active* as well as the *ethical* quality of therapeutic interaction, where the therapist and the family share a mutual responsibility for shaping and influencing the nature of the interactions. In this way, it involves more complexity than the orientation of an individual that arises from mindfulness practices, and is more explicitly intersubjective (i.e., involving interaction between different subjects).

This relational orientation of family therapy is congruent with those psychotherapy models that describe therapeutic interaction as coinciding with a mindfulness-based intersubjectivity between clients and practitioner. For instance, in writing about her mindfulness-based therapy with children, Goodman (2005) suggests that psychotherapeutic presence "refers to more than being in the physical company of another person. It refers to a felt sense of being with another, of *mindfulness-in-connection*" (p. 199). This mindfulness-in-connection is grounded in a "quality of mind" or mindful orientation of the therapist that "involves being aware of the fluctuations of our own attention while we are emotionally engaged with a patient" (p. 201). However, one's awareness as a practitioner is not centered solely upon oneself, but "must sit somewhere between therapist and client" (quoted in Goodman, p. 201), a relational understanding of mindfulness that is similar to dialogic family therapy.

Surrey (2005) provides a detailed account of relational mindfulness in her overview of relational psychotherapy, echoing the teaching of Buddhist master Thich Nhat Hanh (1998) regarding mindfulness as an awareness of relationality. Nhat Hanh refers to mindfulness as "looking deeply" and noting the interrelationships and connections between objects in their "dependent co-arising," thereby cultivating an enhanced relational orientation in the world (p. 59). Similarly, Surrey describes relational psychotherapy as a "process whereby the therapist and the patient are working with the intention to deepen awareness of the present relational experience, with acceptance" (p. 92). In this approach, the dominant notions of "self" and "individuality," taken for granted as the key elements of emotional health are challenged and replaced by a more relational framework where "connection is described as the core of psychological well-being and is the essential quality of growth-fostering and healing relationships" (p. 92). Such an intersubjective orientation in dialogic family therapy would be a sine qua non for the emergence of relational mindfulness.

Attitudes and Ethics of Therapeutic Relationship

Therapists using dialogic approaches to family therapy have explored the qualities of responsive relationship and the attitudinal stance that is needed as a foundation for facilitating dialogic interaction. For instance, in their consideration of the existential states that render a person or family resilient to illness, Griffith and Griffith (2002) have developed an inventory of qualities that foster resilience on a physical, personal, and relational level: hope, agency, purpose, communion, gratitude, and joy (p. 268). All of these attitudinal postures in family therapy are reminiscent of the attributes of relational presence that Surrey (2005) identifies as critical for the therapist to cultivate in the therapeutic relationship in mindfulness-based psychotherapy, and that include "sustained empathic attentiveness, responsiveness, and openness to joining and to being moved in the relationship, as well as an attitude of respect, inquiry, care, and humility" (p. 93).

In *Full Catastrophe Living*, Kabat-Zinn (1990) described attitudinal foundation of mindfulness practice as comprising these specific elements: nonjudging, patience, beginner's mind, trust, nonstriving, acceptance, and letting go (pp. 33–40; see also Kabat-Zinn, 2005, p. 102). The Buddhist nun Pema Chodron (1997) summarizes the expression of mindfulness in an interpersonal context as consisting of compassion, respect, and "do no harm" (pp. 32). She writes, "The ground of not causing harm is mindfulness, a sense of clear seeing with respect and compassion for what it is we see. . . . Mindfulness is the ground; refraining is the path" (pp. 32–33). There are intriguing differences between some of the specific qualities in these lists that may reflect the different cultural contexts from which they have emerged. For instance, "beginner's mind" and nonstriving suggest a Buddhist background, compared with hope in dialogic approaches (Griffith & Griffith, 1994, 2002), which echoes a more Christian sensibility. However, both mindfulness and dialogic family therapy highlight an attitudinal foundation in the posture of the practitioner as being critical to the emergence of the relationality and mindfulness.

Relational Notion of the Self

The most intriguing parallel between family therapy that draws on systems thinking and mindfulness practices that draw on the Buddhist idea of *anatta*, or no-self, is the fact that both have coalesced much of their conceptual thinking around the notion of the relational self. Rather than conceptualizing the self as an isolated, independent entity or an individual separate "I" disconnected from the world, family therapists redeveloped the notion of the self into a more *relational* construct. Tomm (1998b) writes that with "respect to the self, social constructionists emphasize the view that our sense of self is generated through the conversations about ourselves in which we are embedded. Relationships are not just the passive outcome of interaction but a proactive process of co-construction depending on how each interactant gives meaning to the events and behaviours taking place" (p. 174). In dialogic approaches, the focus of therapy is on the interanimating process by which the self and the other are mutually authored in and through conversation. Representations "of the 'other' are contained and located within our 'selves.' In this view, there can be no 'I' without the 'other,' and no 'other' without the 'I,' and it is language that makes this so" (Penn & Frankfurt, 1994, p. 221).

Surrey's (2005) exploration of mindfulness-based psychotherapy bears a resemblance to the growing interest in intersubjectivity in psychotherapy where one's interior realm is constituted through interactions and relationships in the "exterior" world. However, Surrey argues that mindfulness-based relational therapies expand the idea of intersubjectivity into a more encompassing and profoundly relational notion of "interbeing," a word coined by Nhat Hanh to describe the interdependence and interconnection of all existence. In a manner reminiscent of the contextual and relational orientation of family therapists, mindfulness-based therapists facilitate the emergence of a therapeutic context that, according to Surrey, becomes "an exercise of mindful awareness of relationship directed toward the movement of connection and disconnection, and toward the creation of a new, more empathically connected culture within which healing occurs" (p. 96). Such a relationally mindful therapy is transformative of the therapeutic framework itself, for such a reorientation precipitates a "shift from a psychology of entities to a psychology of movement and dialogue. Self, other and the relationship are no longer clearly separated entities but mutually forming processes" (Surrey, 2005, p. 107).

For Kabat-Zinn (2005), the mutuality of presence that constitutes relational mindfulness transcends intersubjectivity and moves into the realm of interbeing, where seeing and "being seen complete a mysterious circuit of reciprocity, a reciprocity of presence" (p. 199). The relational quality of being is a leitmotif that runs through Kabat-Zinn's writings (p. 43), describing how attentiveness strengthens connectedness (p. 121), which is fundamental to our sense of belonging in the world (p. 144). It is this mutuality of presence and profound relationality to each other that link the suffering of individuals or family members to us as therapists: Kabat-Zinn would insist that it is being "in reciprocal relationship to everything makes the suffering of others our suffering" (p. 12).

Cultivation of Dialogic Relationships

Forming dialogic relationships entails the shift from primarily subject–object (I–It) relationships to subject–subject (I–Thou) relationships, a relational posture central not only to dialogic family therapy but to various forms of relational mindfulness in psychotherapy (Surrey, 2005; Goodman, 2005). Surrey describes the subject-to-subject relationship that emerges out of mindfulness in relational therapy, in which clients and therapists come "to this moment of mutuality through the particulars of who we are, therapist-patient, woman-man, I and Thou (Buber, 1970), touching deeply into our most fundamental human connection" (p. 106). Mindful dialogue invites true listening, which in turn extends our ways of knowing and understanding. In contrast, a lack of mindfulness or inattention to both inner and outer experience permits us to divide the self from the other, the "I" from the "Thou," effectively predicating the world on division.

In the creation of a conversational domain in family therapy, each person seeks to move beyond objectifying the other as an Other with no necessary relational connection to oneself. In the dialogic space of therapy, it is hoped that both the client and therapist will strive to maintain themselves and protect each other as subjects. For it is in this attentive and nonjudgmental mutuality of "deep listening" that "each participant is treated as a subject, and the act of responsive listening opens a space for felt meanings" (Penn & Frankfurt, 1994, p. 230). For family therapists, the dialogic quality of I–Thou relationships is a critical and influential perspective that informs the therapeutic interaction by "mapping which regions of one's relationship ecology are marked by decay from I–Thou into I–It relations. This map sets the direction for the therapy. This perspective suggests that we think about the knowledge and skills needed to detect this decay and restore I–Thou relationships" (Griffith & Griffith, 2002, p. 23).

Moving from Monologic Discussion to Dialogic Conversation

Therapists within the dialogic approach to family therapy propose moving from simultaneous monologues that are dominated by a single-voiced perspective to dialogic interaction where there is a multiplicity of voices interanimating and in contact with each other. For Griffith and Griffith (1994), the "creation of a conversational domain is closely related to a shift from monologues to dialogues in conversation" (p. 81). Drawing on Buber, Dostoevsky, and Bakhtin, they insist that dialogic interaction involves "a respectful reflection on multiple perspectives that stand side by side within the same conversation. Out of this speaking, listening, reflecting, a criss-crossing of perspectives arises within which new ideas are born" (p. 81).

In dialogic family therapy, multistressed families are perceived as being embedded in self-contained monologues that anchor conflictual interpersonal patterns of interaction. As conflict becomes more dominant in family interactions, the outer discussion and inner conversations of family members become more rigid, single-voiced, and closed. As the awareness of family members coalesces around these monologues, their responses to each other become increasingly constrained, judgmental, and constricted, given that in a monologic position they "listen to themselves and are unresponsive to others" (Penn & Frankfurt, 1994, p. 223). Through the introduction of reconciling voices that coexist alongside the more negative and judgmental voices, the monologue is relativized and dialogized so that it becomes more multivoiced and nonjudgmentally attentive to others. Dialogue "listens to others and is open, inviting, relative, and endless because it is future-oriented. It awaits an answer" (p. 223).

For Penn (2001), it is through "the discovery of one or more new voices, [that] we become positioned differently to retell the old story, to find a lost one, or to create the beginning of a new one" (p. 47). This re-positioning is grounded in the fact that the "creation of these dialogues contextualizes in advance the reception of negative self-discourse" (Penn & Frankfurt, 1994, p. 219), thereby changing the conversations we have with ourselves. Andersen (2004) describes how each of the voices is given a "home" and how they coexist side by side dialogically "as in every peacework" (p. 223).

This relativizing and contextualizing of monologic "voices" that permits one to reposition oneself bears a suggestive resemblance to the process of "distancing" or "decentering" in the mindfulness-based cognitive therapy described by Segal et al. (2002). As used to prevent depression relapse in their clients, "decentering meant seeing thoughts in a wider perspective, sufficient to be able to see them as simply 'thoughts' rather than necessarily reflecting reality" (p. 39). While dialogic family therapy possesses a greater sensibility to contributing to persons moving from a monologic to a more dialogic stance towards *others* interpersonally through particular therapy practices, mindfulness-based practices also promote a dialogic orientation to the polyphony or multiplicity of "voices" that arise intrapersonally in one's awareness.

Therapeutic Practices

Cultivating Therapeutic Self-Awareness in the Present Moment

As family therapy evolved from a first-order perspective (the therapist acting instrumentally on the family) to a second-order perspective (the family and the therapist interacting within one domain as a family–therapist unit), therapists shifted their awareness to include not only the impact of their own actions upon the family, but the ways in which their responses were being influenced and shaped by the family in mutually responsive, moment-by-moment interactions. For family therapist Karl Tomm (1998b), this shift entailed a commitment "to look at my looking to see what I was seeing and to listen to my listening to hear what I was hearing, [which] constituted a major transformation in my patterns of thinking as a therapist" (p. 177). In his educational guidelines for empowering "self" and "other" in family therapy, Tomm (n.d.) develops an inventory for orienting one's own personal awareness as a practitioner so that one is "looking at one's own looking and listening to one's own listening" as well as "looking at the other's looking and listening to the other's listening." Tomm terms this orientation on the part of the therapist as *recursioning* or as *being mindful*.

For Tom Andersen (1992), being sensitive to and in touch with one's own experiences entails a bodily and sense awareness as well as a more psychological awareness. "When life comes to me, it touches my skin, my eyes, my ears, the bulbs of my tongue, the nostrils of my mouth. As I am open and sensitive to what I see, hear, feel, taste, and smell. I can also notice 'answers' to those touches from myself, as my body, 'from inside,' lets me know in various ways how it thinks about the outside touches" (p. 55; see also Kabat-Zinn, 2005, pp. 185–241, 388–391). Andersen (1997) develops the contours of his awareness as a family therapist further by proposing that his awareness is constituted by an interaction between four ways of knowing: rational, practical, relational, and bodily. He proposes that while all four ways of knowing contribute to a therapist's awareness and provide ongoing orientation, it is the *relational* (how one positions oneself responsively in a relation to another) and *bodily* ways of knowing that are foundational for therapeutic relationships. Bodily knowing "comprises all the micro responses to our being-in-the-world which our five senses and our acts of breathing provide. Bodily knowing contributes to our grasping a felt meaning of the moment, long before that meaning can be formed in words" (p. 126).

Such a therapeutic epistemology is congruent with the microcommunications in mindfulness-based therapy with children (Goodman, 2005), as well as the therapist's awareness of his or her own psychological, relational, and bodily states in relational mindfulness (Surrey, 2005). For instance, in Goodman's (2005) description of her relationship posture with clients, mindfulness practice on the part of a practitioner includes the stance of "not knowing," where one's diagnostic understanding is held "in suspension, so that it [does] not interfere with the task of making an authentic connection" with the client's individuality and experience (p. 203). As with the Buddhist notion of beginner's mind, Goodman insists that holding "our concepts and theories lightly allows us to make a journey of codiscovery with the child" (p. 204), a sentiment echoed by practitioners of dialogic therapy (Pare & Lysack, 2004). Beginner's mind frees the therapist to be attentive to the microcommunications that move responsively between client and therapist. Goodman writes that "a sense of connection and understanding may be the result of a stream of reciprocal perceptions that are too fleeting to track" (p. 206), an observation that is very helpful in family therapy.

In mindfulness-based therapy, the *therapist* continually notices and returns to noticing the changes and differences in his or her *own* sensations, feelings, thoughts, and experiences as well as being attentive to the bodily experiences or "movements" of *clients* (Andersen, 1995). In

Surrey's (2005) approach, therapists augment their awareness by also "attending to the flow of the relationship and the shifting qualities of connection and disconnection, including their energetic, textural, and emotional qualities" (p. 94). As both therapist and client become more deeply and mutually engaged in the therapy as a setting for meditation, it may be deepened into a form of co-meditation practice, where the interpersonal connection and the relational spaces *between* the client and practitioner become the focal point of mindful awareness. As Surrey notes, while "the therapist's focus remains on the experience of the patient, both patient and therapist are engaging in a collaborative process of mutual attentiveness and mindfulness in and through relational joining" (p. 94).

Mindfulness as Attending to What Is Present: Client Bodily States as Language

Both teachers of mindfulness and therapists using dialogic approaches to family therapy emphasize cultivating and deepening one's awareness, or "deep seeing," by being attentive moment by moment to what is present. It is interesting to note that both Kabat-Zinn (2005, p. 390; see also p. 43) and the family therapist Tom Andersen (2004, p. 215) use the identical quote from the philosopher Wittgenstein as an illustration of this orientation. "The aspects of things that are most important for us are hidden because of their simplicity and familiarity. (One is unable to notice something because it is always before your eyes)."

Dialogic family therapists expand their understanding of language beyond merely verbal communication to encompass all semiotic signs and activity in the physical domain. Griffith and Griffith (1994) suggest that in its "biological sense, language exists as a reciprocal signalling through which human mammals coordinate their bodily states, like ships holding formation through the back-and-forth flashing of semaphore flags" (p. 78). In using language to evoke a conversational domain for the sharing of personal stories, therapists guide the conversation by attending to and following the embodied responses of families. Andersen (2004) details the specific practices that he uses in order to respond to the ways in which individuals respond bodily as they share their story (p. 218), directing his attention to small signs and embodied movements (1997, p. 129) in order to actually see the movements and hear what is expressed, rather than searching "behind" or "under" words or gestures (1995, p. 25).

Practitioners responsively select their own posture, language, and interactions, engaging in a physiological tracking and mirroring to enhance the ability of clients to find language in therapy that resonates with their bodily states. "Metaphorically, one can think of this careful modulation of language through following bodily signs as building a linguistic dwelling within which discourse about threatening or painful topics can be safely conducted" (Griffith & Griffith, 1994, p. 87). In an account of her experience in therapy, Melissa Elliott Griffith describes how the embodied responses and actions of a client who was struggling to put a distressing event into words evoked a parallel physiological response sympathetically within her own body. This bodily "resonance" provided a basis for moving through a therapeutic impasse and in a generative direction (p. 89), evoking Jon Kabat-Zinn's image of mindfulness-based therapy as a "friendlier and more self-compassionate way of being in one's body and embracing all of one's thoughts and feelings with acceptance" (2005, p. 437).

Mindful Listening: Witnessing the Suffering of Others

The orientation of family therapy practitioners toward mindful listening when witnessing a person or a family in distress (Gehart & McCollum, 2007), can also be found in the writings of teachers of mindfulness. In family therapy, writes Tomm (1988), "conversations are organized by the desire to relieve mental pain and suffering and to produce healing" (p. 1). And the distinctions that a therapist makes in therapy are those that vector the practitioner in a healing direction, for it "is the therapists' responsibility to be selective in bringing forth distinctions that are therapeutic, in order to orient themselves in a healing direction" (Tomm, 1992, pp. 120, 122).

Penn (2001) suggests that in dialogic approaches to therapy, "listening voice is our primary form of care. The listener is a participant/witness, there to appreciate the whole story of the suffering as many times as it must be told" (p. 43). Penn describes a family therapy session of Tom Andersen's with a couple (two men dying of AIDS), where Andersen's bodily posture was one of attentive, nonjudgmental, moment-by-moment listening. Penn writes, "I had the perception that he was a blank slate expressing his willingness to be written on. He was listening from his center, deep inside the content of what they were saying, to the difficulty they were having anticipating leaving each other" (p. 43). Andersen's responses and questions emerged out of this attentive listening, and facilitated a profound shift in the conversation. Penn writes: "When we began this conversation, our sadness joined us together as islands are joined together under the sea, many of our thoughts almost touching each other. After the question our talk suddenly moved into a celebration of life after death" (p. 43).

Such an emphasis on attentive listening as a form of therapeutic or healing care is also central to Kabat-Zinn's (2005) notion of dialogue. "Learning to listen and participate in conversations with others is the heart of such healing, and of true communication and growing. It is an embodiment of relationality and mutual regard" (p. 449). Such an orientation to cultivating an awareness of and a compassionate response to the suffering of others is also central to the teachings of Thich Nhat Hanh (1995). "When we are mindful, touching deeply the present moment, we can see and listen deeply, and the fruits are always understanding, acceptance, love, and the desire to relieve suffering and bring joy" (p. 14). Nhat Hanh originally developed this form of active mindfulness in the midst of relentless violence, trauma, and suffering among the people of Vietnam. In his meditative community, Buddhist novices were invited "to go out and help people and to do so in mindfulness. We called it engaged Buddhism. Mindfulness must be engaged. Once there is seeing, there must be acting" (p. 91).

LOVINGKINDNESS IN THE THERAPEUTIC RELATIONSHIP

In placing lovingkindness at the center of mindfulness practices, Kabat-Zinn (2005) writes, "Remember that mindfulness practice is a radical act of love. That means that compassion and self-compassion lie at its root" (p. 303). This interest in a notion of lovingkindness as a constituent dimension of the therapeutic relationship is also present in family therapy. For instance, Tomm (1998a) confesses that he finds the notion of the "biology of love as a basis for humanness quite compelling" (p. 137) He writes, "What has been of particular interest to me in Maturana's theory is that he discloses the centrality of love in the evolution of multi-cellular living systems as well as in the evolution of human relationships and culture . . . in which love has been a core generative process" (1998b, p. 185). Drawing on Humberto Maturana's writings, Tomm uses the term "therapeutic love" to describe the ethical posture of the therapist in an empowering relationship with a family (Lysack, 2005, pp. 36–41), a relational stance that is the opposite of "therapeutic violence." Therapeutic violence takes place in therapy when practitioners impose their will or world perspective on the client in any manner. In contrast, therapeutic love entails the therapist opening up an interpersonal space for both parties to exist alongside each other in freedom.

The journeys of teachers of mindfulness and therapists in family therapy converge in many landscapes in their search for relational mindfulness, but they meet in this one territory no less than any other: compassion and the patterns of healing in relationships are both the *mystery* to which we are drawn, and the *pathway* by which we travel. Weingarten (1999) braids these threads together as she writes, "Comfort, care, connection, commitment, and compassion— these are a few of the words in my spiritual lexicon. Listening and love—these are a few of the practices I embrace in my clinical work" (p. 241).

CONCLUSION

In this chapter, I have explored the different ways in which dialogue and compassionate listening can be understood as the external counter- part to the interior cultivation of mindfulness. As a form of positioning in an attentive posture of interaction with clients, relational mindful- ness is enacted in specific micropractices of relationship and forms of moment-by-moment responsivity that encourage healing processes in family relationships. The conceptual resources available in dialogical approaches to working with families can enhance relational mindful- ness in therapy. These theoretical resources include the relational stance of the therapist in the therapeutic relationship, the therapist's attitudes and ethical posture, the relational notion of the self, the cultivation of dialogic relationships, and the movement from monologic discussion to dialogic conversation.

Drawing on these conceptual resources as a framework for mind- fulness-based family therapy, this chapter has provided an overview of the therapeutic practices that can deepen the presence of relational mindfulness in therapy. The foundational practice entails the therapist cultivating awareness of his or her own inner dialogue in the present moment as well as attending to the bodily states of clients as a form of language. In addition, relational mindfulness includes the ability to engage in compassionate listening through witnessing the suffering of others. In all of these instances, these practices are enacted in order to evoke the presence of lovingkindness on the part of both the client and the therapist within a dialogic space, thereby providing a relational con- text for the healing of relationships.

REFERENCES

Anderson, H. (1997). *Conversation, language, and possibilities: A postmodern approach to therapy.* New York: Basic Books.

Andersen, T. (1992). Reflections on reflecting with families. In S. McNamee & K. Gergen (Eds.), *Therapy as social construction* (pp. 54–68). London: Sage.

Andersen, T. (1995). Reflecting processes: Acts of forming and informing. In S. Friedman (Ed.), *The reflecting team in action: Collaborative practice in family therapy* (pp. 1–37). New York: Guilford Press.

Andersen, T. (1997). Researching client–therapist relationships: A collaborative study for informing therapy. *Journal of Systemic Therapies, 16*(2), 125–133.

Andersen, T. (2004). If your pain found a voice what would it say?: Psychotherapy as collaboration. *Human Systems, 15*(4), 213–226.

Bakhtin, M. (1984). *Problems of Dostoevsky's poetics.* Minneapolis: University of Minnesota Press.

Becvar, D. (2003, September/October). Utilizing spiritual resources as an adjunct to family therapy. *Family Therapy Magazine, 2*(5), 31–33.

Bell, L. G. (1998). Start with meditation. In T. Nelson & T. Trepper (Eds.), *101 interventions in family therapy* (Vol. 2, pp. 52–56). New York: Haworth Press.

Chodron, P. (1997). *When things fall apart.* Boston: Shambhala.

Fulton, P. (2005). Mindfulness as clinical training. In C. Germer, R. Siegel, & P. Fulton (Eds.), *Mindfulness and psychotherapy* (pp. 55–72). New York: Guilford Press.

Gehart, D., & McCollum, E. (2007). Engaging suffering: Towards a mindful re-visioning of family therapy practice. *Journal of Marital and Family Therapy, 33*(2), 214–226.

Germer, C. (2005). Teaching mindfulness in therapy. In C. Germer, R. Siegel, & P. Fulton (Eds.), *Mindfulness and psychotherapy* (pp. 113–129). New York: Guilford Press.

Germer, C., Siegel, R., & Fulton, P. (2005). *Mindfulness and psychotherapy.* New York: Guilford Press.

Goodman, T. (2005). Working with children: Beginner's mind. In C. Germer, R. Siegel, & P. Fulton (Eds.), *Mindfulness and psychotherapy* (pp. 197–219). New York: Guilford Press.

Griffith, J., & Griffith, M. (1994). *The body speaks: Therapeutic dialogues for mind–body problems.* New York: HarperCollins.

Griffith, J., & Griffith, M. E. (2002). *Encountering the sacred in psychotherapy.* New York: Guilford Press.

Hayes, S., Follette, V., & Linehan, M. (Eds.). (2004). *Mindfulness and acceptance: Expanding the cognitive-behavioral tradition.* New York: Guilford Press.

Kabat-Zinn, J. (1990). *Full catastrophe living: Using the wisdom of your body and mind to face stress, pain, and illness.* New York: Delta Paperbacks.

Kabat-Zinn, J. (2005). *Coming to our senses: Healing ourselves and the world through mindfulness.* New York: Hyperion.

Lysack, M. (2002). From monologue to dialogue in families: Internalized other interviewing and Mikhail Bakhtin. *Sciences pastorales/Pastoral Sciences, 21*(2), 219–244.

Lysack, M. (2003). "When the sacred shows through": Narratives and reflecting teams in counsellor education. *Sciences pastorales/Pastoral Sciences, 22*(1), 115–146.

Lysack, M. (2005). Empowerment as an ethical and relational stance: Some ideas for a framework for responsive practices. *Canadian Social Work Review, 22*(1), 31–51.

Morgan, W., & Morgan, S. (2005). Cultivating attention and empathy. In C. Germer, R.

Siegel, & P. Fulton (Eds.), *Mindfulness and psychotherapy* (pp. 73–90). New York: Guilford Press.

Nhat Hanh, T. (1995). *Living Buddha, living Christ.* New York: Riverhead Books.

Nhat Hanh, T. (1998). *The heart of the Buddha's teaching: Transforming suffering into peace, joy, and liberation.* Berkeley, CA: Parallax Press.

Pare, D., & Lysack, M. (2004). The willow and the oak: From monologue to dialogue in the scaffolding of therapeutic conversations. *Journal of Systemic Therapies, 23*(1), 6–20.

Penn, P. (2001). Chronic illness: Trauma, language, and writing: Breaking the silence. *Family Process, 40*(1), 33–52.

Penn, P., & Frankfurt, M. (1994). Creating a participant text: Writing, multiple voices, narrative multiplicity. *Family Process, 33*(3), 217–231.

Rosenthal, J. (1990, September/October). The meditative therapist. *Family Therapy Networker, 14*(5), 38–41, 70–71.

Schwartz, R. (1999). Releasing the soul: Psychotherapy as a spiritual practice. In F. Walsh (Ed.), *Spiritual resources in family therapy* (pp. 223–239). New York: Guilford Press.

Segal, Z., Williams, J. M., & Teasdale, J. (2002). *Mindfulness-based cognitive therapy for depression: A new approach to preventing relapse.* New York: Guilford Press.

Simon, D. (1996). Crafting consciousness through form: Solution-focused therapy as a spiritual path. In S. Miller, M. Hubble, & B. Duncan (Eds.), *Handbook of solution-focused brief therapy* (pp. 44–62). San Francisco: Jossey-Bass.

Simon, R. (1999). Don't just do something, sit there. *Networker, 23*(1), 34–46.

Surrey, J. (2005). Relational psychotherapy, relational mindfulness. In C. Germer, R. Siegel, & P. Fulton (Eds.), *Mindfulness and psychotherapy* (pp. 91–110). New York: Guilford Press.

Tomm, K. (1988). Interventive interviewing: Part III. Intending to ask lineal, circular, strategic, or reflexive questions?" *Family Process, 27*(1), 1–15.

Tomm, K. (1992). Therapeutic distinctions in an on-going therapy. In S. MacNamee & K. Gergen (Eds.), *Therapy as social construction* (pp. 116–135). London: Sage.

Tomm, K. (1998a). Co-constructing responsibility. In S. McNamee & K. Gergen (Eds.), *Relational responsibility* (pp. 129–137). Thousand Oaks, CA: Sage.

Tomm, K. (1998b). Epilogue: Social constructionism in the evolution of family therapy. In J. West, D. Bubenzer, & J. Bitter (Eds.), *Social constructionism in couple and family counseling* (pp. 173–187). Alexandria, VA: American Counseling Association Press.

Tomm, K. (n.d.). *Four guidelines for empowering "self" and "other."* Unpublished handout.

Twemlow, S. (2001a). Training psychotherapists in attributes of "mind" from Zen and psychoanalytic perspectives: 1. Core principles, emptiness, impermanence, and paradox. *American Journal of Psychotherapy, 55*(1), 1–21.

Twemlow, S. (2001b). Training psychotherapists in attributes of "mind" from Zen and psychoanalytic perspectives: 2. Attention, here and now, nonattachment, and compassion. *American Journal of Psychotherapy, 55*(1), 22–39.

Walsh, F. (Ed.). (1999). *Spiritual resources in family therapy.* New York: Guilford Press.

Weingarten, K. (1999). Stretching to meet what's given: Opportunities for a spiritual practice. In F. Walsh (Ed.), *Spiritual resources in family therapy* (pp. 240–255). New York: Guilford Press.

Wylie, M. S., & Simon, R. (2004, November/December). The power of paying attention. *Psychotherapy Networker, 28*(6), 59–67.

IV TEACHING AND LISTENING

How can we go about teaching students and others to listen deeply and be deeply present? For that matter, how can we go about learning this ourselves?

This section opens with the contribution of Shauna Shapiro and Christin Izett, who offer empirical evidence that meditation and mindfulness practices facilitate empathy. They suggest that this may occur through stress reduction (how can I listen to you if I am upset?), increased compassion for self (generalizing to others), and through *reperceiving* (the capacity to perceive what was subject as object). For teachers who wonder how these skills could be taught as part of an education curriculum, Diane Gehart and Eric McCollum describe a mindfulness course they employ with graduate students.

Gregory Kramer and Florence Meleo-Meyer note that mindfulness— whether in meditation or in the midst of daily activities—is generally practiced as a solitary activity. It is not automatically clear how to use such practices in an interpersonal context. They offer the process of Insight Dialogue as a way to bridge this gap.

And finally, Rebecca Shafir describes how she teaches mindfulness and communication in her work as a speech/language neurotherapist. She offers helpful, concrete advice about how to listen more deeply and avoid practices that obstruct the flow of communication.

10 Meditation

A Universal Tool for Cultivating Empathy

SHAUNA L. SHAPIRO
CHRISTIN D. IZETT

Empathy is a well-established construct in psychology, one whose value is prominent across all theoretical orientations. Although it has been studied for hundreds of years, with contributions from philosophy, theology, developmental psychology, social and personality psychology, ethology, and neuroscience, the field suffers from a lack of consensus regarding the nature of this phenomenon. Empathy is defined by Rogers as an "accurate understanding of the [client's] world as seen from the inside. To sense the [client's] private world as if it were your own" (1961, p. 284). He further defines empathy within the therapeutic context as a twofold process. The first component involves the counselor accurately sensing what the client is feeling. The second component involves the counselor's capacity to communicate this sensing to the client in a way that is attuned with the client's current feeling state.

Empathy is generally understood as a multidimensional construct, including affective, cognitive, self-focused, and other focused dimensions (Davis, 1983). Further, empathy is viewed as relational, with intrapersonal and interpersonal components (Bennett, 1995). It has been presented as a necessary condition for effective therapy (Arkowitz, 2002; Rogers, 1992). In fact, according to Bohart and colleagues, "empathy accounts for as much and probably more outcome variance than does specific intervention" (Bohart, Elliott, Greenberg, & Watson, 2002, p. 96).

Yet therapists have been challenged to find ways of cultivating empathy, which may be harder to learn than specific therapy skills and knowledge (Lazarus, 1993). Further, although empathy is heralded as an essential skill of therapy, very little attention has been devoted to finding ways to cultivate empathy in therapist training programs. And in fact, Traux and Carkhuff's (1963) findings suggest that empathy tends to stay the same or decrease among students in formal counseling training programs (Lesh, 1970).

Few empirical studies have inquired into the process of *learning* the essential therapeutic skill of empathy. Our review of the literature yielded only six published studies that have examined the effects of various training modalities on cultivating empathy in therapists in training (Bierman, Carkhuff, & Santilli, 1972; Cutcliffe & Cassedy, 1999; Lesh, 1970; Nerdrum, 1999; Nerdrum, 2002; Shapiro & Walsh, 2007). The discrepancy between the field's valuing of empathy and its relative inattention to finding effective ways of teaching it to therapists in training needs to be addressed. It is time to consciously and creatively explore means of cultivating this vital and universal therapeutic skill.

Meditation practices may be one effective way to do this. Meditative theory suggests that empathy is an essential means for gaining insight into the nature of oneself, others, and the relation between oneself and the rest of the world (Wallace, 2001). Systematic practices to cultivate empathy have been developed and practiced for the past 2,500 years. Western psychology could benefit by exploring how to integrate these practices into training programs.

Meditation is defined as a family of techniques designed to cultivate greater awareness, wisdom, and compassion (Walsh & Shapiro, 2006). Although Western psychology has only touched the surface of how meditation practice can affect empathy, the integration of meditative techniques and Western psychology with the aim of cultivating greater empathy in therapists is potentially of great value. For example, Western psychology emphasizes that a "precondition for empathy to occur is to listen personally with truly interested attention and nonjudging receptivity" (Barrett-Lennard, 1997, p. 108). Specific meditation practices, such as mindfulness practice, train one in the cultivation of this interested attention and nonjudging receptivity. In addition to mindfulness practice, there are detailed meditative practices to explicitly cultivate empathy, lovingkindness, and compassion. Each of these is discussed in more detail below.

This paper briefly reviews the research on meditation and empathy, summarizes current theory on how meditation can aid in cultivating empathy, and finally focuses on specific meditations and processes that may increase empathy and thereby enhance the therapeutic relationship.

RESEARCH: MEDITATION AND EMPATHY

Meditation offers a unique means of cultivating empathy, integrating affective, cognitive, intra-, and interpersonal elements (Beddoe & Murphy, 2004, reviewed below). It is a means for transforming both one's perception and one's relationship to oneself and others. It allows us to recognize and understand our own feelings, providing insight into these same feelings in others (Baillie, 1996; Levenson & Ruef, 1992; Beddoe & Murphy, 2004).

The potential benefits of various forms of meditation in developing empathy have been the focus of empirical inquiry for decades. Keefe (1976) conducted a series of studies examining empathy and its development. He suggested that some varieties of meditation, "especially those derived from Zen traditions, encourage behaviors that facilitate empathy" (Keefe, 1976, p. 13). He concluded that meditation can: (1) increase the capacity to maintain one's focus of attention and awareness upon events of the present moment, (2) increase the ability to keep complex cognitive processes in temporary abeyance, (3) refine sensitivity to one's own emotional responses to another person, and (4) help one to relax and clear one's mind for further work.

In addition, in a sample of 39 master's level students, Lesh (1970) found that counseling psychology students demonstrated significant increases in empathy after Zen meditation intervention compared to a waiting list control group and a group of students who expressed no interest in meditation (Lesh, 1970). Empathy was measured by students' ability to accurately assess emotions expressed by a videotaped client.

A randomized controlled trial examined the effects of an eight-week mindfulness-based stress reduction (MBSR) intervention for medical and premedical students. Seventy-eight students were randomized into the intervention or waiting list control group. Findings indicated significant increases in empathy levels in medical students as compared to controls (Shapiro, Schwartz, & Bonner, 1998). The control group showed similar changes after receiving the MBSR intervention.

A recent study examining the effects of MBSR on counseling psychology students found significant postintervention increases in empathy (Shapiro & Brown, 2007). It extended previous research by examining the process variables involved in the cultivation of empathy, namely mindfulness and self-compassion. Findings immediately following the intervention indicated that MBSR training significantly increased *mindfulness* as measured by the Mindful Attention Awareness Scale (MAAS; Brown & Ryan, 2003), and that increases in mindfulness mediated changes in empathy and self-compassion immediately following the intervention. It is noteworthy that a brief intervention could significantly affect both empathic concern for others as well as compassion for self. The finding that mindfulness intervention increases self-compassion supports previous controlled research demonstrating increases in self-compassion in health care professionals after MBSR intervention (Shapiro, Astin, Bishop, & Cordova, 2005). This ability to relate to oneself with compassion and empathy could lead to the ability to relate to others, including one's patients, with compassion and empathy. We speculate that self-compassion is related to the development of empathy for others, and discuss this theory below.

THEORIES: HOW MEDITATION CULTIVATES EMPATHY

What are the psychological processes that allow us to be empathic? And how does meditation practice facilitate this capacity? We suggest three pathways by which meditation cultivates empathy: (1) reducing stress, (2) increasing self-compassion, and (3) learning to disidentify with one's own subjective perspective.

Reducing Stress

It has been shown that when people are distressed their empathy levels *decrease* (Galantino, Baime, Maguire, Szapary, & Farrar, 2005). "In humans, fear and distress lead to self-directed efforts, and, thus, are prohibitive of empathy" (Eisenberg et al., 1994).

Larson (1993) describes stress as interpersonal in nature, but states that its origins are rooted in relationship to ourselves. He argues that people, especially helping professionals, place unrealistic expectations on themselves ("It is up to me to help this person, I must alleviate their pain"). This can be a major source of intrapersonal stress. "Questioning ourselves and the work we do is inevitable . . . but blame and guilt can . . . undermine your well-being and your ability to care" (Larson, 1993, p. 65).

Galantino and colleagues (2005) examined the effect stress has on empathy by observing changes in salivary cortisol levels (an index of stress in the body). They did this in conjunction with various scales measuring mood, burnout, and empathy levels in health care professionals before and after a mindfulness meditation training program. The results indicate that participants experienced heightened levels of negative affect and lower levels of empathy as a function of cortisol levels in the body.

A similar study of baccalaureate nursing students explored the effects of an 8-week MBSR course on stress and empathy. The MBSR course was intended to provide students with methods for coping with personal and professional stress and to "foster empathy through intrapersonal knowing" (Beddoe & Murphy, 2004). Differences in the pretest and posttest measures of anxiety indicated that participation in the intervention significantly reduced students' anxiety. Favorable trends were observed in a number of stress dimensions including attitude, time pressure, and total stress. Two dimensions of empathy, personal distress and fantasy (the tendency to identify with fictional character's experience), also demonstrated favorable trends. Both studies indicate that there is an inverse relationship between stress and empathy.

Therapists commonly experience "compassion fatigue" (Figley, 2002; Weiss, 2004) due to the emotional stress that is often a part of therapeutic work. Stress can reduce providers' ability to establish strong relationships with patients (Enochs & Etzbach, 2004; Renjilian, Baum, & Landry, 1998), ostensibly by decreasing empathy. Thus, practices designed to teach stress management skills to therapists in training may represent a form of "preventive treatment" for individuals at risk for burnout and decreased empathy.

Meditation-based interventions have been shown to significantly decrease stress in a wide range of clinical and nonclinical populations (for review see Baer, 2003). Research has specifically demonstrated significant decreases anxiety, stress, and depression in health care professionals, and students in training (Shapiro et al., 1998, 2005). Therefore, meditation-based intervention may help cultivate empathy simply by reducing one's stress. Research by Shapiro and colleagues lends preliminary evidence to this hypothesis. Their path model analysis of MBSR intervention for medical students demonstrates that decreases in stress and anxiety mediate increases in empathic concern for others (Shapiro et al., 1998). This finding supports earlier research (Lesh, 1970) demonstrating that reducing anxiety through meditation-based intervention increases empathy levels.

Self-Compassion and Empathy

Researchers have hypothesized that the cultivation of self-compassion is related to empathic concern for others. Self-compassion involves an awareness that you are suffering and a genuine care and kindness for yourself to end that suffering (Neff, Kirkpatrick, & Rude, 2007). This connection and care for oneself is related to an understanding and care for others. As Barrett-Lennard (1997) states, "self empathy opens the way to interpersonal empathy" (1997, p. 111). Gendlin (1974) argues that interpersonal empathy emerges from self-directed empathy. Research demonstrates that therapists who lack self-compassion and are critical and controlling toward themselves are also more critical and controlling toward their patients and have worse patient outcomes (Henry, Strupp, Butler, Schacht, & Binder, 1993).

Meditation may also help cultivate empathy by teaching self-empathy or self-compassion. Meditative traditions specifically teach that empathy which excludes empathy for oneself is incomplete (Kornfield, 1993). The practices instruct us to infuse our awareness with qualities of kindness, nonjudgmentalness, and acceptance. Relating to ourselves in this way, moment by moment, facilitates a more compassionate relationship to ourselves and our experiences (Shapiro & Schwartz, 2000). We are comfortable with our own internal experiences, and therefore able to bring greater sensitivity and care to others' internal experiences. Put another way, "the person who is at home with the subjective stirrings of his or her own inner being tends to be sensitive to the inner felt world of others and is not afraid of responding from this awareness" (Barrett-Lennard, 1997, p. 111).

Rand (2004) suggests that meditation practices that cultivate self-empathy also help facilitate the presence and attention of a therapist toward clients. By being more present to ourselves, we become more embodied and less dissociated. When we are more present in this way, we also become more present to others, and more capable of engaging in a helping, healing relationship. Rand suggests that meditation helps counselors become aware of transference and countertransference that may arise in the therapeutic relationship, and that this awareness makes therapy more likely to be successful.

The research on MBSR for counseling psychology students noted above (Shapiro & Brown, 2007) supports this hypothesis. Findings indicated that MBSR increased students' levels of self-compassion and that these increases were related to increases in empathic concern for others (Shapiro & Brown, 2007).

Reperceiving and Empathy

Finally, learning to take the perspective of another is an essential part of cultivating empathy. When we are able to disidentify with own perspective and shift to seeing that of another person we are able to experience greater empathy. Meditation practice trains us to know what our own experience is so that we do not project our feelings onto the client. As Lesh puts it, "projection occurs [when] the supposed perceiver sees in the other person what he, the perceiver, is feeling, but is unaware of in himself" (1970, p. 66). Meditation practice cultivates this ability to clearly distinguish between our own feelings and that of the client, creating the space for true empathy to arise.

Further, meditation practice trains us to not only know what we are feeling as we are feeling it, but to relate to it in a different way. Mindfulness cultivates the ability to shift our perspective beyond our own personal, subjective experience, a process termed *reperceiving* (Shapiro, Carlson, Astin, & Freedman, 2006). Through this process we are able to disidentify from the contents of consciousness (i.e., our thoughts) and view our moment-by-moment experience with greater clarity and objectivity. Rather than being immersed in the drama of our personal narrative or life story, we are able to stand back and simply witness it. This allows space for us to also witness and see clearly what someone else is feeling. When we are not so caught up in ourselves we create room to attend to another. As Kristeller and Johnson (2005) write, "This loosening of attachment to self may facilitate an ability to experience the needs of others" (p. 401).

As described by Shapiro and colleagues (2006):

> Reperceiving can be described as a rotation in consciousness in which what was previously "subject" becomes "object." This shift in perspective (making what was subject, object) has been heralded by developmental psychologists as key to development and growth across the lifespan (Kegan, 1982). . . . Mindfulness is simply a continuation of the naturally occurring human developmental process whereby one gains an increasing capacity for objectivity about one's own internal experience. (p. 6)

Reperceiving is a natural developmental process that can be illustrated with an example: A mother of two sons, ages 8 and 3, is celebrating her birthday. For the special occasion, each child decides to give his mother a gift. Her 8-year-old gives her some flowers from their garden and her 3-year-old gives her one of his toys. While each gift is age appropriate, the 3-year-old's gift illustrates how a child of this age is caught in his own self-centered (i.e., egocentric) perspective and cannot see his mother's desires. His world is largely subjective, simply an extension of himself. As a result, he cannot interpret the subjective experiences, perspectives, or desires of another. As he grows in cognitive capacity, he will experience an increased ability to take the perspective of others (e.g., maybe my mother has different desires from mine). This new developmental capacity allows what was previously subjective to be seen objectively. This shift can be viewed as the dawning of empathy, an awareness of another's separate and unique needs, desires, and perspectives.

As Shapiro and colleagues note (2006):

> Reperceiving, in which there is increasing capacity for objectivity in relationship to one's internal/external experience, is in many ways the hallmark of mindfulness practice. Through the process of intentionally focusing nonjudgmental attention on the contents of consciousness, the mindfulness practitioner begins to strengthen what Deikman refers to as "the observing self" (Deikman, 1982). To the extent that we are able to observe the contents of consciousness, we are no longer completely embedded in or fused with such content. For example, if we are able to see *it*, than we are no longer merely *it*; i.e., we must be *more* than *it*. Whether the *it* is pain, depression, or fear, reperceiving allows one to dis-identify from thoughts, emotions, body sensations as they arise, and simply be with them instead of being defined (i.e., controlled, conditioned, determined) by them. Through reperceiving one realizes, "this pain is not me," "this depression is not me," "these thoughts are not me," as a result of being able to observe them from a meta-perspective. (p. 6)

The shift in perspective we are describing is analogous to our earlier example of the 3-year-old who over time is eventually able to see himself as separate from the objective world in which he had previously been embedded. However, in this case, the disidentification is from the content of one's mind (thoughts, feelings, self-concepts, memories). Through reperceiving there is a profound shift in one's relationship to thoughts and emotions, the result being greater clarity and perspective.

As events arise in the mind, they are simply noted, as opposed to eliciting an automatic or unconscious reaction. This is very helpful in cultivating empathy for another person. As we develop this equanimity, we are able to meet even the deepest and strongest emotions in ourselves and our clients without having to solve them, fix them, or react to them. We can simply empathize with them.

As meditation practice deepens, this developmental shift of perspective continues, leading to a realization that subject and object are not separate but one. The nondual nature of things becomes apparent, and one realizes there is no separation between self and other. A Hindu saying eloquently captures this development:

> When I forget who I am I serve you
> Through serving I remember who I am
> And know that I am you.

METHODS AND PROCESS FOR CULTIVATING EMPATHY

How can we bring meditation practices into clinical training programs? What are some specific methods and exercises designed to cultivate empathy and self-compassion? Below we highlight three types of meditation practices that could be introduced into training programs to help cultivate empathy.

Mindfulness Meditation Practices

Mindfulness meditation practice involves bringing a nonjudgmental, curious attention to all of one's experiences as they arise moment by moment. It involves the careful observation and consideration of the body, feelings, mental states, and mental objects of oneself and of others (Wallace, 2001, p. 5). As Wallace (2001) eloquently observes:

> A common theme to each of these four applications of mindfulness is first considering these elements of one's own being, then attending to these same phenomena in others, and finally shifting one's attention back and forth between self and others. Especially in this final phase of practice, one engages in what has recently been called reiterated empathy, in which one imaginatively views one's own psychophysical processes from a 'second-person' perspective. That is, I view my body and mind from what I imagine to be your perspective, so that I begin to sense my own presence not only 'from within' but 'from without.' Such

practice leads to the insight that the second-person perspective on one's own being is just as 'real' as the first-person perspective; and neither exists independently of the other. (p. 5)

Formal mindfulness practices include sitting meditation, body scan meditation, mindful movement, and walking meditation. All of these practices are based on the core instructions to attend to whatever arises with curiosity, openness, and compassion. Sitting meditation involves resting in a comfortable seated position and attending, without judgment, to whatever arises in one's field of consciousness moment by moment. The body scan meditation involves lying on the ground and systematically attending to each part of the body in an open and non-judgmental way. Mindful movement and walking meditations involve bringing this same precise yet relaxed awareness to the moment to moment process of moving.

Lovingkindness (Metta) Meditation

Lovingkindness meditation involves focused aspirations for the well-being of self and others. The lovingkindess meditation helps one become vividly aware of the other person's joys and sorrows, hopes and fears (Wallace, 2001). In traditional Buddhist practice one first cultivates lovingkindness for oneself (Salzberg, 1995). Learning to love and have compassion for oneself is an essential teaching in Buddhism. The Buddha taught that you can search the whole world and not find someone more deserving of your love than yourself. In the next phase of practice one brings to mind someone who is loved and respected and sends the phrases of lovingkindness to them. The circle of lovingkindness continues to expand, first including a dear friend, a neutral person, and finally a "difficult" person. As Wallace (2001) states, "The aim of the practice is to gradually experience the same degree of loving kindness for all people. In this way, the barriers between self and other are gradually broken down and unconditional loving kindness may be experienced" (p. 7). (For basic instructions see *dharma.ncf.ca/introduction/instructions/metta.html*.)

Compassion (Karuna) Meditation

Compassion meditation practice involves the aspiration that one may be free from suffering and its causes. It is closely linked with loving-kindness, where the intention is that others may find genuine happiness and the causes of happiness. In compassion practice, one attends first to someone who is suffering, wishing "May you be free from suffering" or "May your suffering decrease." As one progresses in this practice, one sequentially focuses on oneself, someone in pain, a dear person, a neutral person, and finally on someone for whom one has felt aversion. This practice, like *metta* practice can help to cultivate empathy by breaking down "the barriers separating these different types of individuals until one's compassion extends equally to all beings" (Wallace, 2001, p. 11). Another form of compassion meditation is called Tonglen, a practice involving breathing in the suffering of others and breathing out relief. For example, if your dear friend is in pain, you would breath in her pain and the wish to relieve her pain, and as you breathe out you send her happiness, joy, or whatever she needs to relieve her pain (for basic instructions see *www.shambhala.org/teachers/pema/tonglen1.php*).

It is important to note that Buddhism teaches these practices not as a substitute for service to others but as essential mental preparation for service. This preparation, according to Wallace (2001), "raises the likelihood of such outer behavior being truly an expression of an inner, benevolent concern for others' wellbeing" (p. 12). This seems to be a very helpful model for training students going into the helping profession and clinical work.

Informal Practice: Mindfulness in Daily Life

Although we believe that meditation practices serve to facilitate empathy, we also believe it is important to incorporate exercises and dialogue to accompany the specific practices and to help make explicit the intention of cultivating empathy. It may be important to include exercises to help students bring the insights gained during meditation practice into relationship and interpersonal interactions.

Informal mindfulness practices can help facilitate this deeper understanding. Informal practice involves bringing mindful awareness to whatever one is engaged in moment by moment. For example, *listening* can be an informal mindfulness practice. Intentionally attending to what another person is saying is a mindfulness practice, although it is not a formal meditation practice. A mindful listening exercise that we use in the graduate course for counseling psychology students is to introduce the definition of mindfulness and then practice "intentionally attending to hearing in an open and nonjudgmental way." All persons in the class are invited to share one thing currently causing stress in their lives, and one thing for which they are grateful. They are invited to notice emotions, thoughts, body sensations, connections to others, questions, and judgments that arise moment by moment during this exercise. Through this exercise we practice mindfully listening to ourselves and each other. Students are invited to let go of what they are going to say and simply be present so that they can fully listen to their classmates. They are invited to trust that when their turn comes they will know what to say in that moment. Students report feeling a deep connection with others and a greater ability to empathize with each other. They are able to notice when their mind is judging or has wandered off and are able to refocus and simply be present for another's experience. Our shared human experience arises as we truly hear both the pain and the joys that we all face.

A second informal mindfulness practice that we use to help cultivate empathy is a mindful dialogue explicitly about what opens and closes the doorway to empathy. Small groups of students (three to four) spend 10 minutes in a mindful dialogue with the intention of exploring insights gained during formal meditation practice and discussing how these insights apply to intra- and interpersonal empathy. Explicitly linking the relationship between self-care and care for others is emphasized. For example, attention is focused on the traditional instructions of the lovingkindness meditation, which begins with oneself before expanding to include loved ones and eventually all beings.

A third informal mindfulness practice involves mindfully reading and listening to poetry. Mindful readings of poetry from different cultures and spiritual traditions can be used to present universal human themes (Shapiro, 2001). These poetry readings can help students see things from different perspectives, gain a sense of interconnectedness, and understand paradox.

CONCLUSION

Future research can help elucidate the numerous questions that arise in determining how to incorporate meditation into clinical training. For example, randomized clinical trails are needed to determine what kinds of practices will be most effective for cultivating empathy (e.g., mindfulness meditation or lovingkindness meditation?). It will also be important to determine when in a therapist's clinical training these practices can be most effectively introduced and in what format.

It will also be helpful to explore whether meditation practice is enough to clinically increase empathy in meaningful ways, or if it is necessary to explicitly cultivate empathy by engaging in specific informal practices to help translate the insights gained during practice into clinically meaningful empathy. For example, will developing a mindfulness meditation practice cultivate an ability to empathize with others and to skillfully communicate this understanding to others, or are explicit informal listening and dialoguing practices needed? It will be important to compare formal meditation training with interventions that blend formal practice with informal exercises explicitly targeting empathy.

Although this area of inquiry is still in its infancy, evidence suggests that meditation practices allow for significant transformations in one's relationship to self and other, which lead to increased empathy. Meditation may be a universal tool for cultivating empathy, and thus the integration of meditation into clinical training programs merits further exploration.

REFERENCES

Arkowitz, H. (2002). An integrative approach to psychotherapy based on common processes of change. In J. Lebow (Ed.), *Comprehensive handbook of psychotherapy*. New York: Wiley.

Baer, R. (2003). Mindfulness training as a clinical intervention: A conceptual and empirical review. *Clinical Psychology: Science and Practice, 10*, 125–143.

Baillie, B. (1996). A phenomenological study of the nature of empathy. *Journal of Advanced Nursing, 2*, 1300–1308.

Barrett-Leonard, G. T. (1997). Recovery of empathy: Toward self and others. In A. C. Bohart & L. S. Greenberg (Eds.), *Empathy reconsidered: New directions in psychotherapy* (pp. 312–334). Washington, DC: American Psychological Association.

Beddoe, A., & Murphy, S. (2004). Does mindfulness decrease stress and foster empathy among nursing students? *Journal of Nursing Education, 43*, 305–312.

Bennett, J. A. (1995). Methodological notes on empathy: Further considerations. *Advances in Nursing Science, 18*, 36–50.

Bierman, R., Carkhuff, R., & Santilli, M. (1972). Efficacy of empathic communication training groups for inner city preschool teachers and family workers. *Journal of Applied Behavioral Science, 8*, 188–202.

Bohart, A. C., Elliott, R., Greenberg, L. S., & Watson, J. C. (2002). Empathy. In J. C. Norcross (Ed.), *Psychotherapy relationships that work: Therapist contributions and responsiveness to patients*. Oxford, UK: Oxford University Press.

Bohart, A. C., & Greenberg, L. S. (1997). Empathy in psychotherapy: An introductory overview. In A. C. Bohart & L. S. Greenberg (Eds.), *Empathy reconsidered: New directions in psychotherapy*. Washington, DC: American Psychological Association.

Brown, K. W., & Ryan, R. M. (2003). The benefits of being present: Mindfulness and its role in psychological well-being. *Journal of Personality and Social Psychology, 84*, 822–848.

Cutcliffe, J., & Cassedy, P. (1999). The development of empathy in students on a short, skills based counseling course: A pilot study. *Nursing Education Today, 19*, 250–257.

Davis, M. H. (1983). Measuring individual differences in empathy: Evidence for a multidimensional approach. *Journal of Personality and Social Psychology, 44*, 113–126.

Eisenberg, N., Fabes, R. A., Murphy, B., Karbon, M., Maszk, P., Smith, M., et al. (1994). The relations of emotionality and regulation to dispositional and situational empathy-related responding. *Journal of Personality and Social Psychology, 66*, 776–797.

Enochs, W. K., & Etzbach, C. A. (2004). Impaired student counselors: Ethical and legal considerations for the family. *Family Journal, 12*, 396–400.

Figley, C. R. (2002). Compassion fatigue: Psychotherapists' chronic lack of self-care. *Journal of Clinical Psychology, 58*, 1433–1441.

Galantino, M. L., Baime, M., Maguire, M., Szapary, P. O., & Farrar, J. T. (2005). Association of psychological and physiological measures of stress in health-care professionals during an 8-week mindfulness meditation program: Mindfulness in practice. *Stress and Health: Journal of the International Society for the Investigation of Stress, 21*, 255–261.

Gendlin, E. T. (1974). Client-centered and experiential therapy. In D. A. Wexler & L. N. Rice (Eds.), *Innovations in client-centered therapy* (pp. 24–41). New York: Wiley.

Henry, W. P., Strupp, H. H., Butler, S. F., Schacht, T. E., & Binder, J. L. (1993). The effects of training in time-limited dynamic psychotherapy: Changes in therapist behavior. *Journal of Consulting and Clinical Psychology, 61*, 434–440.

Keefe, T. (1976). Empathy: The critical skill. *Social Work, 21*, 10–14.

Kornfield, J. (1993). *A path with heart: A guide through the perils and promises of spiritual life.* New York: Bantam Doubleday Dell.

Kristeller, J. L., & Johnson, T. (2005). Cultivating lovingkindness: A two-stage model of the effects of meditation on empathy, compassion and altruism. *Journal of Religion and Science, 40*, 391–408.

Larson, D. G. (1993). *The helper's journey: Working with people facing grief, loss, and life-threatening illness.* Champaign, IL: Research Press.

Lazarus, R. S. (1993). Coping theory and research: Past, present, and future. *Psychosomatic Medicine, 55*, 234–247.

Lesh, T. V. (1970). Zen meditation and the development of empathy in counselors. *Journal of Humanistic Psychology, 10*, 39–74.

Levenson, R. W., & Ruef, A. M. (1992). Empathy: A physiological substrate. *Journal of Personality and Social Psychology, 63*, 234–246.

Merton, T. (Ed. & Trans.). (1965). *The way of Chuang Tzu.* New York: New Directions.

Neff, K. D., Kirkpatrick, K., & Rude, S. S. (2007). Self-compassion and its link to adaptive psychological functioning. *Journal of Research in Personality, 41*, 139–154.

Nerdrum, P. (1999). Maintenance of the effect of training in communication skills: A controlled follow-up study of level of communicated empathy. *British Journal of Social Work, 27*, 705–722.

Nerdrum, P. (2002). The trainees' perspective: A qualitative study of learning empathic communication in Norway. *Counseling Psychologist, 30*, 609–629.

Rand, M. L. (2004). Vicarious trauma and the Buddhist doctrine of suffering. *Annals of the American Psychotherapy Association, 7*, 40–41.

Renjilian, D. A., Baum, R. E., & Landry, S. L. (1998). Psychotherapist burnout: Can college students see the signs? *Journal of College Student Psychotherapy, 13*, 39–48.

Rogers, C. R. (1961). *On becoming a person: A therapist's view of psychotherapy.* Boston: Houghton Mifflin.

Rogers, C. R. (1992). The necessary and sufficient conditions of therapeutic personality change. *Journal of Consulting and Clinical Psychology, 60,* 827–832.

Salzberg, S. (1995). *Loving-kindness: The revolutionary art of happiness.* Boston: Shambhala.

Shapiro, S. (2001). Poetry, mindfulness, and medicine. *Family Medicine, 33,* 505–506.

Shapiro, S. L., Astin, J., Bishop, S., & Cordova, M. (2005) Mindfulness-based stress reduction and health care professionals. *International Journal of Stress Management, 12,* 164–176.

Shapiro, S. L., & Brown, K. (2007). *Mindfulness and empathy.* Unpublished manuscript.

Shapiro, S. L., Carlson, L., Astin, J., & Freedman, B. (2006). Mechanisms of mindfulness. *Journal of Clinical Psychology, 62,* 373–386.

Shapiro, S. L., & Schwartz, G. E. (2000). Intentional systemic mindfulness: An integrative model for self-regulation and health. *Advances in Mind-Body Medicine, 16,* 128–134.

Shapiro, S. L., Schwartz, G., & Bonner, G. (1998). Effects of mindfulness-based stress reduction on medical and premedical students. *Journal of Behavioral Medicine, 21,* 581–599.

Shapiro, S. L., & Walsh, R. (2007). The farther reaches. In T. Plante & C. Thoresen (Eds.), *Spirit, science and health: How the spiritual mind fuels the body* (pp. 57–71). Westport, CT: Praeger/Greenwood.

Traux, C. B., & Carkhuff, R. R. (1963). For better or worse: The process of psychotherapeutic personality change. In C. B. Traux (Ed.), *Recent advances in the study of behavior change.* Montreal, Canada: McGill University Press.

Wallace, A. (2001). Intersubjectivity in Indo-Tibetan Buddhism. *Journal of Consciousness Studies, 8,* 209–230.

Walsh, R., & Shapiro, S. L. (2006). The meeting of meditative disciplines and Western psychology: A mutually enriching dialogue. *American Psychologist, 61,* 227–239.

Weiss, L. (2004). *Therapist's guide to self-care.* New York: Brunner/Routledge.

11 Inviting Therapeutic Presence

A Mindfulness-Based Approach

DIANE GEHART
ERIC E. MCCOLLUM

Beneath the concerns about managed care, empirical support, diagnosis, and theoretical orientation, psychotherapy remains an encounter between two (or more) people whose primary shared goal is improvement in the life circumstances of clients and how they relate to those circumstances, both externally and internally. While the goals of therapy may range from simple and concrete problem solving to more broad-ranging growth and development, outcome studies indicate that the quality of the therapist–client relationship is an important ingredient in this work, although there are various opinions about its degree of importance. Lambert (1992), for instance, suggested that fully 30% of outcome variance was accounted for by the relationship between therapist and client. In a meta-analytic study, Martin, Garske, and Davis (2000) report a much more conservative finding of about 5%. No one, however, suggests that the therapeutic relationship has no importance in the practice of psychotherapy (Bachelor & Horvath, 1999; see also Lambert & Simon, Chapter 2, this volume). But what does the therapist offer the client in the therapy relationship that leads to successful outcomes? Much of the training on this issue is couched in terms of therapist skills and actions—for instance, reflective listening, "joining," or attending (e.g., Young, 2005). However, some suggest that a more ineffable quality—*therapeutic presence*—is a primary ingredient of a sound and nurturing therapeutic relationship (Geller & Greenberg, 2002; McDonough-Means, Kreitzer, & Bell, 2004).

Because therapeutic presence is more a quality of relationship than a set of skills—a state of *being* rather than a state of *doing*, in other words—it is harder to bring formally into training programs. In training, attention to therapists' ways of being most often occurs under the rubric of exploring and developing the "self of the therapist." Exercises in this area typically focus on trainees understanding their own family of origin experiences, personal emotional triggers, and relationship style preferences, the impact of difficult life events, and how these personal characteristics intersect with the process and content of therapy (Horne, 1999; Timm & Blow, 1999). Some approaches are model specific; they apply the same therapy model to the trainee's experience that is used in work with clients. Thus, psychoanalysts are psychoanalyzed (Bibring, 1954), and Bowen family systems therapists engage in efforts to differentiate in their own families (Bowen, 1978). Other approaches do not rely on a specific therapeutic model but promote trainees' examination of their life experiences in general. Using this model, a trainee might be helped to understand the ongoing emotional vestiges of a parental divorce, for instance, learning how and when these become obstacles in therapy and what to do to minimize their impact. This process aims to increase therapeutic presence by removing the obstacles to it rather than by promoting or examining it directly. Few direct approaches to developing therapeutic presence are described in the literature, however. We suggest that mindfulness meditation (*vipassana*) and other contemplative practices have the potential to help trainees develop therapeutic presence directly, not just through the process of removing constraints on presence (which remains important) but by helping trainees directly cultivate the qualities of being in the present that are basic to therapeutic presence.

In this chapter, we describe the mindfulness-based curriculum we developed for teaching new marriage and family therapists how to develop therapeutic presence in their early clinical coursework. The curriculum was implemented in practicum courses during the students' first clinical work with clients and was based on existing mindfulness-based therapies, such as mindfulness-based stress reduction (MBSR; Kabat-Zinn, 1990) and mindfulness-based cognitive therapy (MBCT; Segal, Williams, & Teasdale, 2001) as well as our professional and personal experiences with mindfulness and other Buddhist practices.

DEFINING THERAPEUTIC PRESENCE

Therapeutic presence is most commonly defined as the quality of self or way of being that therapists bring to the therapeutic encounter (Geller & Greenberg, 2002). This quality of self is considered to have intrapersonal, interpersonal, and transpersonal elements, including elements of empathy, compassion, charisma, spirituality, transpersonal communication, patient responsiveness, optimism, and expectancies, making it elusive and difficult to operationalize (McDonough-Means et al., 2004). Therapists are routinely trained to "build rapport," "be empathetic," or "join" with a client using skills such as reflecting feelings, summarizing, and refraining from advice giving (Young, 2005). Although useful, these techniques focus more on the *content* of the therapist's communication than the therapist's "being" or presence in the room. Therefore, for the purpose of this discussion, it is important to emphasize that we are focusing on the *quality of being* rather than a set of rapport-building or joining skills, which may or may not facilitate this quality of being. Specifically, we see therapeutic presence as the attitude or stance toward present experience that the therapist brings to the moment-to-moment therapeutic encounter. In Buddhist terms, this stance is characterized by *wisdom*—the ability to see experience clearly—as well as *compassion*, the deep understanding of our common suffering as humans and how that unites us (Brach, 2003). Thus, the unvarnished apprehension of the present moment with all its joys and difficulties is cradled in our common humanity to prevent it from becoming either coldly objective or arising as a barrier between us. Therapist and client play different roles in the encounter but remain human throughout.

Bugenthal (1987), an existential–humanistic therapist, describes three components of therapeutic presence: being open and available to all parts of the client's experience, being open to all of one's own experience as one is with the client, and being able to respond from the immediacy of that experience. From this perspective, the therapist must be able to fully encounter the client's experience while maintaining the ability to observe his or her own reactions and experiences and to act thoughtfully based on the confluence of these aspects of the relationship. The following vignette, observed by one of us (EM), illustrates these components of therapeutic presence in action. At one point, about midway through the therapy hour, a therapist said to her client, "I've noticed that both times you told me you were feeling that you weren't living up to what I might be expecting of you as a client happened when my mind was wandering a bit. I wonder if you aren't exquisitely sensitive to others' connection to you and, when it seems distant, assume that you have done something wrong." Clearly this therapist was able to attend equally to her client and herself and suggest meaning from a consideration of both domains. Thus, she was fully present to both her own experience and that of the client, a hallmark of what we define as therapeutic presence.

We suggest that therapeutic presence comprises a quality of being that a therapist brings to the therapeutic relationship/encounter that actively promotes and facilitates the therapeutic process and goal attainment, and that:

- is not necessarily related to specific verbalizations or techniques (e.g., empathetic statements, open-ended questions, etc.) but rather is experienced more as a stance or orientation to the experience of the present moment.
- involves the whole person of the therapist: physical, emotional, cognitive, social, and spiritual.
- is generally characterized by a balanced expression of engaged compassion and equanimity (Salzburg, 1995), recognizing that both joy and suffering are part of the human journey.
- is further expressed by the ability to attend openly and clearly both to one's own experience and the client's experience, and to act therapeutically from the immediacy of that attention.

THERAPEUTIC PRESENCE AND THERAPIST TRAINING

No mental health discipline has developed a systematic approach for teaching therapeutic presence as a skill or ability. As noted above, it has remained an elusive quality that emerges from personal growth work, which typically takes the form of personal psychotherapy, either as part of the supervision process or via a referral for treatment outside the training environment (Geller & Greenberg, 2002). More specifically, within our field of family therapy, training has primarily focused on case conceptualization and intervention skills (the "doing" mode) rather than the person of the therapist (the "being" mode), with the two major exceptions being intergenerational and experiential therapies (Simon, 2006). This focus on conceptualization and skill development has led to highly refined and technical models of supervision that are largely unprecedented in psychotherapy. The introduction of common factors research (Sprenkle & Blow, 2004; Hubble, Duncan, & Miller,

1999), which attributes 30% of positive outcome in therapy to the quality of the therapeutic relationship, has ignited greater interest about how the self of the therapist affects therapeutic outcome.

The broadening of focus from technique to relationship is also happening in the field of medicine. Medical practitioners have argued that the Buddhist meditation practice of mindfulness can be used to develop greater "healing presence" for doctors and nurses (Epstein, 2003a, 2003b; McDonough-Means et al., 2004). One study demonstrated that mindfulness was effective for reducing medical students' stress and increasing their empathy (Shapiro, Schwartz, & Bonner, 1998), and another demonstrated how mindfulness could be used to reduce nurses' burnout (Cohen-Katz et al., 2005). Based on recent neurological findings on brain functioning, Siegel (2007) has suggested that the part of the brain that is developed in the process of the emotional attunement that characterizes secure attachment is the same part of the brain that is developed during mindfulness practice, thus providing a biological explanation for how mindfulness practice can improve the quality of intra- as well as interpersonal interactions.

Within the field of psychotherapy, Geller and Greenberg's (2002) qualitative study of therapeutic presence included the finding that meditation practices such as mindfulness are commonly cited as a means for developing therapeutic presence. Anecdotally, trainers in marriage and family therapy (MFT) and counseling are experimenting with mindfulness to help new therapists more successfully cope with the high levels of anxiety associated with the early stages of MFT training (e.g., Germer, Siegel, & Fulton, 2005) and counseling (Newsome, Christopher, Dahlen, & Christopher, 2006).

Considered from a biological perspective, mindfulness training is likely to improve a therapist's quality of presence as well as overall ability to implement the knowledge he or she has acquired by studying. Studies on mindfulness indicate that mindfulness practice increases a person's capacity to regulate mood and increases positive affect (Davidson et al., 2003) by increasing the ability to use the prefrontal cortex (the reason centers of the brain) to shut down stress responses from the limbic system and the fight-flight-freeze mechanism. This allows one to more readily calm oneself and access reason in moments of stress. Clearly, this ability would be useful for the stress that therapists in training face as they begin to see clients. If trainees increase their ability to calm their stress reactions, they will be more likely to draw readily on their knowledge and training.

WHAT IS MINDFULNESS MEDITATION?

Mindfulness meditation is most closely associated with Buddhism, which, in various sutras (sacred texts), has provided the most in-depth description of the practice and its effects. However, one need not be a Buddhist or ascribe to Buddhist or any other particular spiritual beliefs in order to practice and profit from mindfulness meditation (see Batchelor, 1998). Other religions include similar practices. For instance, centering prayer in the Christian tradition has many similarities to Buddhist mindfulness meditation (Keating, 2006). Goleman (1996) provides an overview of the meditative practices of many of the world's spiritual traditions.

As mindfulness meditation has been adapted for use in psychotherapy, scholars have begun to examine its structure and process apart from a particular religious or spiritual context. Bishop and colleagues (2004) suggest that mindfulness comprises two components—self-regulation of attention and a particular orientation to one's experiences. Self-regulation consists of a purposeful focus of one's attention on immediate, present experience, typically physical sensations and mental events. Thus, the mindfulness practitioner attempts to carefully observe experience *in the present, as it occurs*. Mindfulness is therefore distinguishable from a common approach to therapy training—reflection—which one considers one's experience in retrospect. The second component of mindfulness proposed by Bishop and colleagues is the particular orientation toward experience that the practitioner adopts. This orientation is one of "curiosity, openness and acceptance" (p. 232). Rather than trying to control, suppress, or promote various thoughts, emotions, and other aspects of experience, mindfulness practice invites the practitioner to approach all experience as it arises with a sense of exploration and welcome so that it can be examined carefully and investigated. Thus, a practitioner might not try to distract herself from the pain of a headache during meditation but rather turn with curiosity to the pain—considering such things as its location, intensity, quality, and shape.

Taken together, these two components of mindfulness increase one's ability to more closely and accurately observe what one is feeling, thinking and sensing without becoming absorbed in it. Mindfulness is not unlike the experience of watching a movie—we periodically pull back and realize that the story we have become absorbed in is simply a story represented by light and sound in a theater. When practiced over time, mindfulness helps develop our ability to pull back and observe the process of experience, and not simply engage with its content.

The parallels between mindfulness and our view of therapeutic presence are what led us to consider using mindfulness meditation as an invitation to therapeutic presence for our students. Therapeutic presence requires clearly attending to both one's own and the client's experience while holding that attention in a context of compassion. These are precisely the skills that mindfulness meditation teaches. Furthermore, meditation allows beginning students to become familiar with the process of self-observation in an environment less stress ridden than initial clinical interviews. Finally, it helps to balance the "doing" mode so common to marriage and family therapy models that stress action and intervention with the "being" mode that we take to be crucial for being present with clients. Eric McCollum tells his students that formal meditation practice is like working out at the gym. The workout is not the end in itself. One works out in order to take the gains made in the gym out into the world to pursue valued activities. In the case of mindfulness and therapy, we meditate in order to become better observers of our own experience and to learn to hold that experience with compassion. We then try to bring that same presence to the therapeutic encounter.

INVITING THERAPEUTIC PRESENCE INTO THE CLASSROOM

As our awareness, understanding, and personal practice of mindfulness have grown, so has our interest in using it to help therapist trainees cultivate therapeutic presence. Both of us being teachers, there is a temptation to *teach* our students to be more therapeutically present. This, of course, flies in the face of what we should be doing: trying to create an environment of learning to *be* rather than to *do*. We have come, therefore, to think of ourselves as *inviting* our students to engage in the process of therapeutic presence. The invitation is for them to become curious about their own experience in a context we have tried to make as safe and supportive as we can. The mechanism for this effort has been introducing them to mindfulness meditation and other contemplative practices.

We developed a curriculum that fit within our programs, both master's programs in marriage and family therapy, one accredited by the Commission for Accreditation of Marriage and Family Therapy Education (COAMFTE) and the other by the Commission for the Accreditation of Counseling and Related Programs (CACREP). Both of our universities are public institutions, neither having a tradition of integrating spirituality into its curriculum. For this reason, we were sensitive to the need for respecting the diversity of students' religious perspectives and traditions. Thus we chose to use the terms *contemplative* as well as *mindfulness*, with the former preferred in Judeo–Christian contexts and the latter by Buddhists and the scientific community.

The curriculum was designed to fit within two-semester practicum courses required for the degree at each institution. These practicum courses were centered around students' first clinical experiences. In one program, all clients were seen at the university clinic; at the other, students were all placed in community fieldwork settings. Both courses had additional content requirements that attended to student needs in beginning clinical placements, such as writing case notes, treatment planning, crisis management, and working with site supervisors.

Curriculum Overview

Mindfulness was introduced in multiple ways with emphasis on experiential learning and a deemphasis on academic knowledge. We began by providing a rationale for teaching new therapists mindfulness meditation. We had to provide some reason for teaching the practice of meditation to students who had signed on to learn the practice of therapy! We used much of the material presented above to make the link between therapeutic presence and mindfulness. Without it, the meditation practice might seem extraneous or tangential to the primary reasons students were in the class—to learn to be marriage and family therapists. Once this groundwork had been laid, we used a variety of teaching methods and learning activities, including:

- Regular outside mindfulness practice by students
- Written journals
- Practice logs
- Readings
- In class lectures
- In class discussions
- In class meditations (guided and nonguided)

Outside Mindfulness Practice

As part of the course, students were expected to engage in a minimum of 5 minutes of contemplative practice 5 days a week; students were encouraged to do more if they found it helpful. This was a target that students were free to exceed; they were informed that they would not be penalized with a lower grade for failing to meet the target each week. Instead their grades were based on the *quality* of the reflections in their weekly journals (see below). Although this 5-minute requirement is minimal, we believed it was a fair expectation given the academic, work, and personal demands in our students' lives. Many students reported that because this requirement sounded reasonable, they were more successful than they had been in the past with establishing a daily meditation routine. In fact, most students frequently exceeded the 5-minute, 5-day minimum.

Meditation Journal

Each week students completed a journal entry reflecting on their mindfulness or contemplative practice for the week. We gave students a list of prompts to help focus their journal entries:

- Were you able to practice for at least 5 minutes five times in the week? If so, what helped you achieve this goal? If not, what were the impediments?
- Describe your mindfulness or contemplative practice (focus, etc.)
- Describe strategies you used for returning to your focus. Were you able to be patient with yourself during the practice?
- Describe any insights you may have gained from observing your mind.
- Describe any differences in your daily life that may have resulted from this practice.
- Describe any differences in your professional practice that may have resulted from this practice.
- Describe new insights, practices, or experiences related to developing therapeutic presence.

We collected and read the journals at several points throughout this semester. This allowed us to closely monitor students' experiences and modify the curriculum as needed. Many students reported that journaling helped them to make links between mindfulness and the development of therapeutic presence. Several students reported that journaling was very helpful for the first 8 weeks or so of class, when it helped them reflect on what worked and what did not. After students had found a way to successfully and regularly integrate a contemplative practice into their daily routine, the journals then became more of a distraction from the practice. Therefore, we developed the option of using a practice log instead.

Practice Logs

In addition to and/or instead of journals, students completed daily (Figure 11.1) or weekly (Figure 11.2) logs of their mindfulness practice. These logs are designed to help students keep track of their practice by noticing what strategies helped them create time to practice, the effects of different mindfulness foci (if they used more than one), and any effects in their daily lives. The weekly log is designed to help motivate by creating a sense of accomplishment on one hand (regular practice is quite noticeable) and accountability on the other (lack of practice is equally apparent). The logs were especially helpful for students who had hectic lives and who found such a tool motivating.

Readings

Instructors have numerous options for assigned readings on mindfulness and contemplative practices. We chose the following:

- *The Zen of Listening* (Shafir, 2000)
- *Meditation for Dummies*, 2nd edition (Bodin, 2006)[1]

Shafir (2000) provided an excellent description of how mindfulness applies to listening, thus addressing one of the most basic therapeutic skills and therefore highly applicable in students' work and the course goal of developing therapeutic presence. Bodin (2006) provided a comprehensive introduction to a range of meditation and contemplative practices without privileging a specific religious tradition. Thus, students could develop a form of practice that fit with their personal beliefs, whether within a formal tradition or otherwise.

In-Class Lectures and Discussion

The contemplative curriculum was added as a 5- to 30-minute class segment at the end or beginning of the weekly 3-hour class meeting. The placing of the mindfulness activity was a challenge. Beginning with

FIGURE 11.1. Mindfulness practice daily log. Copyright 2007 by Diane R. Gehart, PhD. Reprinted by permission.

Date: Day of Week: M T W Th F S Su   Time: Length of Practice:

General Notes:

Getting to It: What strategies (time of day, place, timers, etc.) made it easiest to practice today?

Quality of Practice: What strategies (type of focus, refocus technique, etc.) helped you to improve the quality of your practice?

Changes in Daily Life: Did you notice any benefits in your daily life (patience, calmness, etc.) from your practice today?

Plans for Next Time: What is one thing you can do later this week to improve practice and/or maximize benefits?

FIGURE 11.2. Mindfulness practice weekly log. Copyright 2007 by Diane R. Gehart, PhD. Reprinted by permission.

Week of: _____   Target # of Days/Time: _____

Mon	Tues	Wed	Thurs	Fri	Sat	Sun
☐ 5 min	☐ 5 min	☐ 5 min	☐ 5 min	☐ 5 min	☐ 5 min	☐ 5 min
☐ 10 min	☐ 10 min	☐ 10 min	☐ 10 min	☐ 10 min	☐ 10 min	☐ 10 min
☐ 20 min	☐ 20 min	☐ 20 min	☐ 20 min	☐ 20 min	☐ 20 min	☐ 20 min
☐ _____	☐ _____	☐ _____	☐ _____	☐ _____	☐ _____	☐ _____
☐ Day off	☐ Day off	☐ Day off	☐ Day off	☐ Day off	☐ Day off	☐ Day off
Note:	Note:	Note:	Note:	Note:	Note:	Note:

Getting to It: *What strategies (time of day, place, timers, etc.) made it easiest to practice this week?*

Quality of Practice: *What strategies (type of focus, refocus technique, etc.) helped you to improve the quality of your practice?*

Changes in Daily Life: *Did you notice any benefits in your daily life (patience, calmness, etc.) from your practice this week?*

Plans for Next Week: *What is one thing you can do next week to improve practice and/or maximize benefits?*

mindfulness helped transition students from outside activity to the class, but it was sometimes difficult to either settle students down enough to focus or, alternatively, gear them up to focus on more academic or clinical tasks afterwards. Ending the class with mindfulness was appealing because it provided a relaxing transition to everyday life; however, it required better time and content management for the rest of the class time. After experimenting with both options, we found that beginning the class with mindfulness was more effective because it was easier to balance it with the rest of the curriculum.

Lectures were kept to a minimum and focused on providing an introduction to mindfulness and contemplative practices, linking them directly to the cultivation of therapeutic presence in students' clinical work. We usually began the mindfulness segment of class with a guided meditation or 5 minutes of group breath meditation without guidance. Afterwards, we allowed time for a lecture and/or discussion of students' experiences and questions. These sessions covered content information about the readings and about mindfulness more broadly, as well as intimate discussions about students' practices and the effect on their personal and professional lives. For example, one day a student shared how a client had become very hostile and aggressive during a session; he began to react by becoming fearful. However, he said he was able to calm this fearful response by just telling himself, "breathe," which he claims he could not have done without practicing mindfulness regularly. Another student shared how he had begun to ask his partner to sit for 5 minutes doing mindfulness meditation after they arrived home from work; he said that their level of conflict greatly diminished on the nights they did this.

These discussions also generated ideas about how to use mindfulness within the context of the students' training. For example, through the group discussions, the idea emerged that doing a short mindfulness practice before seeing clients may help one to be more present with clients in the hours to follow, just as doing mindfulness at the beginning of class was changing the classroom dynamic by increasing students' ability to focus and be present. Thus, the group discussions became a place to share strategies, success stories, and frustrations about their practices.

In-Class Meditations

Numerous meditations were used during class to help teach contemplative practices that would help students develop therapeutic presence.

Three classic mindfulness meditations were used early in the semester to introduce basic mindfulness principles:

- Mindful breath meditation
- Mindful eating meditation
- Mindful walking meditation

In addition to teaching mindfulness using breath as the focus, we included eating and walking meditations with the intention of demonstrating how mindfulness can be used with different stimuli and activities. We found that eating and walking meditation were less threatening to those new to mindfulness and actually served as an excellent preparatory experience before introducing mindful breath meditation.

Ice Meditation

Eric McCollum was first introduced to ice meditation by Dr. Sonja Batten in a workshop on doing acceptance and commitment therapy, which includes many mindfulness techniques (personal communication, May 19, 2006). This exercise provides a way for participants to practice turning attention toward painful or difficult experiences. The participants are each given a small ice cube and asked to hold it in their hand as it melts. They are further invited to observe and be curious about the experience of holding the ice—both physical sensations as well as cognitive and emotional reactions. Holding an ice cube in one's hand quickly produces a number of typically unpleasant results. The cold hurts. The dripping water is messy. One's hand movement is limited for the period of time it takes the ice to melt. Participants are encouraged to simply observe their sensations and reactions—including aversion to the unpleasant experience, the wish to pull away, and impatience with the exercise (e.g., "this is silly") as well as curiosity about the painful feelings, any changes or variations in them that one can sense, the actual feeling of a drop of water dripping from one's hand, and so forth. Time is given for participants to share and discuss what they have observed and how this might relate to ways they can deal with the inevitable unpleasant experiences one will have as a therapist.

Tonglen: Compassion Meditation

Tonglen is a form of Tibetan Buddhist compassion meditation (Brach, 2003). Tonglen takes the opposite approach to the common psychotherapeutic techniques in which a person breathes out their stress and breathes in relaxation. Instead, the practitioner does the reverse: breathes in the sorrow and suffering of others and breathes out blessings and good will. This generosity of spirit underlies the spiritual roots of this Tibetan practice. This meditation exercise is ideal for teaching therapeutic presence because it helps students learn how to remain open in the face of client suffering rather than quickly fix or minimize a client's pain due to their own discomfort.

To teach this meditation, we begin by explaining its roots, the boddhisattva tradition in Mahayana Buddhism in which practitioners take vows to remain in samsara (the cycle of rebirth) until all living beings have reached enlightenment. The focus for those who have taken the vow is to work toward alleviating the suffering of others, hence they are willing to "transform" the suffering of others, which is symbolized in the breathing in of suffering and the breathing out of blessing. Students are then guided to imagine doing this with

- A neutral acquaintance, someone they do not have particularly positive or negative feelings for.
- A loved one, someone the person has strong feelings for.
- An enemy, someone the person has strong negative feelings for.
- A client the student is working with.

Two to three minutes are allowed for the neutral person, visualizing breathing in suffering and breathing out blessings, before moving on to the next person; again, several minutes are allowed for the loved one before moving on to the final two.

Compassion Meditation: Day in the Life

One of the meditations Diane Gehart has used with students was adapted from a meditation led by Jack Kornfield at the 2004 Sacred Art of Healing Conference. This is an extremely intense and intimate guided meditation that has produced the most dramatic immediate responses from students and professional audiences. This meditation is designed to help the participants generate compassion for their meditation partner by imaging the sum total of the joys and sorrows this person will experience over the course of his or her life. Participants are guided through a series of images and asked to apply them to their partner, thus making it a very personal experience. At the same time, the instructions refer to global experiences, thus directing attention to the universality of suffering and joy that characterizes all human lives. This meditation is extremely moving for most students, and many will tear up. Due to the intensity of this exercise, it is only done once in a semester and at least half an hour is allowed for it.

To set up the meditation, Gehart puts students in groups of two and has them face their chairs toward each other. They are instructed to maintain eye contact without staring, allowing the natural flow of focusing on the other then looking away to occur without judgment of self or other.

The meditation begins by having students imagine the joys and difficulties their partner may have experienced throughout the day. Students can be instructed to "imagine the possible stresses" that their partner experienced, such as getting up late, getting a troubling phone call, hitting heavy traffic, or having an argument with a significant other, as well as possible joys, such as waking up with a sense of excitement, receiving good news in the mail, having success with a client, or seeing a child smile their way.

Next, they are asked to broaden their imaginings to possible joys and difficulties that may be going on in the person's life at the moment, such as school stress, relationship problems, ill parents, financial problems, health issues, graduation, a new career, meaningful relationships, dreams fulfilled, and so forth.

After addressing the present, participants are instructed to imagine the birth of their partner and how that birth may have been celebrated or not by those in the child's life. Then participants imagine the struggles and joys of their partner's childhood: first ice cream, being teased at school, riding a bike, being sick, first date, and so forth.

Finally, participants are asked to imagine their partner on their deathbeds: perhaps surrounded by loved ones, perhaps not. Additionally, they are asked to imagine as this person reviews his or her life, what it meant to them and others. Once the meditation is over, students first debrief in pairs and then as a whole group.

CONCLUSION

Integrating contemplative and mindfulness practices into a practicum experience included both academic and experiential elements, such as readings, class discussion, in-class contemplative exercises, and at-home meditation practice. We developed the curriculum to teach therapeutic presence, perhaps one of the most critical, yet elusive qualities of a skilled clinician. Mindfulness, the practice of being fully present and accepting of the moment, provides a unique focused activity to cultivate therapeutic presence, the ability to be fully present with clients.

Students reported that the curriculum achieved its goal and also had other significant effects on their lives. Not only did they report a significant improvement in their ability to be fully present with clients, but they also reported numerous other positive changes in their personal lives. For instance, as they began to see the many resistances they experienced to meditating daily—despite the fact that they nearly uniformly described meditation as helpful to them—they began to understand how clients might find it difficult to change quickly some of the problems they bring to therapy.

Our students also noticed how quickly anxiety led them to become overly involved in their inner experience, usually at the expense of being present with the client. And they began to glimpse the depth of inner criticism that most of us live with—how much we attempt to avoid unwanted parts of our experience and the suffering this strategy causes. They reported that they better understood what it meant and felt like to be present therapeutically, and their comments and in-class behavior provided evidence that a significant shift was happening. Perhaps most important, as our students examined their own experience, they began to have more compassion for their clients—a growing realization that we all share common hopes for happiness and for relief from suffering.

NOTE

1. Despite the potentially off-putting title, our students found this book very helpful. While not a scholarly text, it provides solid information about meditation techniques and experiences.

REFERENCES

Bachelor, A., & Horvath, A. (1999). The therapeutic relationship. In M. A. Hubble, B. L. Duncan, & S. D. Miller (Eds.), *The heart and soul of change: What works in therapy* (pp. 133–178). Washington, DC: American Psychological Association.

Batchelor, S. (1998). *Buddhism without beliefs.* New York: Riverhead Books.

Bibring, G. L. (1954). The training analysis and its place in psycho-analytic training. *International Journal of Psycho-Analysis, 35,* 169–173.

Bishop, S. R., Lau, M., Shapiro, S., Carlson, L., Anderson, N. D., Carmody, J., et al. (2004). Mindfulness: A proposed operational definition. *Clinical Psychology: Science and Practice, 11,* 230–241.

Bodin, S. (2006). *Meditation for dummies* (2nd ed.). New York: Wiley.

Bowen, M. (1978). *Family therapy in clinical practice.* New York: Jason Aronson.

Brach, T. (2003). *Radical acceptance: Embracing your life with the heart of a Buddha.* New York: Bantam.

Bugenthal, J. F. T. (1987). *The art of the psychotherapist: How to develop the skills that take psychotherapy beyond science.* New York: Norton.

Cohen-Katz, J., Wiley, S. D., Capuano, T., Baker, D. M., Kimmel, S., & Shapiro, S. (2005). The effects of mindfulness-based stress reduction on nurse stress and burnout, Part II: A qualitative and quantitative study. *Holistic Nurse Practitioner, 19,* 26–35.

Davidson, R. J., Kabat-Zinn, J., Schumacher, J., Rosenkranz, M., Muller, D., Santorelli, S. F., et al. (2003). Alterations in brain and immune function produced by mindfulness meditation. *Psychosomatic Medicine, 65,* 564–570.

Epstein, R. (2003a). Mindful practice in action: 1. Technical competence, evidence-based medicine, and relationship-centered care. *Families, Systems & Health, 21,* 1–9.

Epstein, R. (2003b). Mindful practice in action: 2. Cultivating habits of mind. *Families, Systems & Health, 21,* 11–17.

Geller, S. M., & Greenberg, L. S. (2002). Therapeutic presence: Therapists' experience of presence in the psychotherapy encounter. *Person-Centered and Experiential Psychotherapies, 1,* 71–86.

Germer, C. K., Siegel, R. D., & Fulton, P. R. (Eds.). (2005). *Mindfulness and psychotherapy.* New York: Guilford Press.

Goleman, D. (1996). *The meditative mind: The varieties of meditative experience.* New York: Tarcher.

Horne, K. B. (1999). The relationship of the self of the therapist to therapy process and outcome: Are some questions better left unanswered? *Contemporary Family Therapy, 21,* 385–403.

Hubble, M. A., Duncan, B. L., & Miller, S. D. (1999) *The heart and soul of change: What works in therapy.* Washington, DC: American Psychological Association.

Kabat-Zinn, J. (1990). *Full catastrophe living: Using the wisdom of your body and mind to face stress, pain, and illness.* New York: Delta.

Keating, T. (2006). *Open mind open heart: The contemplative dimension of the gospel.* New York: Continuum.

Lambert, M. J. (1992). Implications of outcome research for psychotherapy integration. In J. C. Norcross & M. R. Goldstein (Eds.), *Handbook of psychotherapy integration* (pp. 94–129). New York: Basic Books.

Martin, D. J., Garske, J. P., & Davis, M. K. (2000). Relation of the therapeutic alliance with outcome and other variables: A meta-analytic review. *Journal of Consulting and Clinical Psychology, 68,* 438–450.

McDonough-Means, S. I., Kreitzer, M. J., & Bell, I. R. (2004). Fostering a healing presence and investigating its mediators. *Journal of Alternative and Complementary Medicine, 10,* S25–S41.

Newsome, S., Christopher, J. C., Dahlen, P., & Christopher, S. (2006). Teaching counselors self-care through mindfulness practices. *Teachers College Record, 108,* 1881–1900.

Salzburg, S. (1995). *Loving kindness: The revolutionary art of happiness.* Boston: Shambala.

Segal, Z. V., Williams, J. M. G., & Teasdale, J. D. (2001). *Mindfulness-based cognitive therapy for depression: A new approach to preventing relapse.* New York: Guilford Press.

Shafir, R. Z. (2000). *The Zen of listening.* Wheaton, IL: Quest Books.

Shapiro, S., Schwartz, G. E., & Bonner, G. (1998). Effects of mindfulness-based stress reduction on medical and premedical students. *Journal of Behavioral Medicine, 21,* 581–599.

Siegel, D. J. (2007). *The mindful brain: Reflection and attunement in the cultivation of well-being*. New York: Norton.

Simon, G. M. (2006). The heart of the matter: A proposal for placing the self of the therapist at the center of family therapy research and training. *Family Process, 45,* 331–344.

Sprenkle, D. H., & Blow, A. J. (2004). Common factors and our sacred models. *Journal of Marital and Family Therapy, 30,* 113–130.

Timm, T. M., & Blow, A. J. (1999). Self-of-the-therapist work: A balance between removing restraints and identifying resources. *Contemporary Family Therapy, 21,* 331–351.

Young, M. (2005). *Learning the art of helping: Building blocks and techniques* (3rd ed.). Upper Saddle River, NJ: Pearson.

12 Cultivating Mindfulness in Relationship

*Insight Dialogue and the
Interpersonal Mindfulness Program*

GREGORY KRAMER
FLORENCE MELEO-MEYER
MARTHA LEE TURNER

Humans are inherently relational beings; human interactions carry enormous power to hurt or to heal. Even in therapy—that is, in relationships guided by finely honed methods intended specifically to foster healing—the outcome has been shown to depend mostly upon the character and quality of the therapist–client relationship (see Lambert & Simon, Chapter 2, this volume).

Yet the disciplines that train therapists—medicine, psychology, social work—have generally succeeded better at teaching theories, concepts, and techniques of therapy than at fostering the quality of therapeutic relationship. To borrow Nasrudin's famous parable, this situation is reminiscent of looking for one's lost keys where the light is good, rather than looking for them in the place where one dropped them. That is, we continue refining the elements we know how to refine, even though they don't show the highest correlation with outcomes, while we give less attention to the element that most influences outcome, the therapeutic relationship itself—perhaps because we haven't quite seen how to address it.

The meditative practices that are roughly grouped under the heading of mindfulness are able to address this training gap in important ways. That is the thesis of this book, and we heartily agree. Teaching therapists and therapist trainees such forms of meditation is almost guaranteed to help them become more self-aware, more accepting and reflective, more available to the client in the present moment, and more able to choose their responses skillfully.

Nevertheless, while basic mindfulness meditation is able to improve the quality of the therapist–client relationship, it has a limitation parallel to that of the academic helping disciplines. Traditional meditation techniques like those discussed by Steven Hick in Chapter 1 of this volume have sought to develop mindfulness either in solitary formal meditation or in informal situations that are not interpersonal. Examples of formal (or "extraordinary") meditation are meditating alone at a set-aside time or meditating on retreat in a room full of others with whom one carefully avoids interaction. Remembering to be mindful while dressing or brushing one's teeth is an example of informal (or "ordinary") meditation, as is the use of some stimulus in the environment, like red traffic lights or the sound of a passing train, to recall one to inner recollection. Most approaches to meditation stay within these nonrelational options. Moreover, traditional individual meditation can sometimes reify the sense of an isolated and autonomous self, though this is not its intention. When this happens, it is difficult to connect meditation to everyday life or to therapeutic practice.

Searching in solitude for the key to the demands of a particularly challenging type of relationship bears some resemblance to Nasrudin's quandary. It relies on the premise that new habits and responses developed in private meditation will reappear spontaneously in the heat of interactions with other people. This transfer works well enough that solitary meditation has unmistakable benefits for human interactions. But as social beings, humans find interactions with each other uniquely distracting—and uniquely challenging. While most can develop some measure of tranquility, mindfulness, and compassion in solitude, transferring these gains into the give-and-take of real-time human interactions is a second, largely unsupported, challenge.

Because Insight Dialogue (ID) is a formal practice of dialogic meditation, it supports this challenge directly. Based in *vipassana* or insight meditation practices, ID is revolutionary in that it breaks the paradigm of individual, private meditation by cultivating mindfulness while in relationship. Engaging in disciplined, mindful dialogue with one or more other people is the form of this meditation practice—just as sitting or walking, attending to the breath or to the body, are the forms of other practices. In interpersonal meditation we are able to observe our relational hungers (cravings) in real time. We are able to see how suffering arises with those hungers. We learn to support each other, and to be supported, in releasing those hungers.

The benefits of interpersonal meditation transfer easily into everyday life with others. The stimuli offered by everyday interactions are not so different from the stimuli that have been worked with in meditative practice. New skills and habits learned in meditative practice are already adapted to the challenges of relationship. Because of these differences, ID can foster changes in the quality of relationships—including the therapeutic relationship—much more directly than solitary approaches to the cultivation of mindfulness.

The first section of this chapter describes in some detail what ID looks like and how it works. ID exists in a number of forms—retreat practice, weekly groups, online dialogue (both real-time and asynchronous), and in an important offshoot, the Interpersonal Mindfulness Program (IMP). This program, modeled loosely on the Mindfulness Based Stress Reduction program (MBSR), presents the basics of ID in a structured course designed to be accessible to people with no background or interest in the Buddhist roots of ID. Although the IMP presents the same ID practice, its history and norms have developed differently.

After considering the nature of the practice, we will examine how specific orientations and qualities needed in the therapeutic relationship are fostered in ID. As we shall see, the guidelines and contemplations of ID support greater therapist self-awareness and acceptance of dysphoric experience, greater presence to and acceptance of the client, and provide concrete practice in exploring the present moment, with respect and curiosity, with another person.

While ID is an accessible practice that brings important resources to therapist training and the development of the therapeutic relationship, it remains deeply rooted in the larger context of Buddhism. This larger context also has important contributions to make to the practice of therapy. At the simplest level, Buddhism can be considered as a sophisticated psychology, tested over millennia. We give some attention to how this ancient psychology can extend, deepen, and clarify the contemporary secular and Western understandings of mindfulness.

A variety of options for learning and practicing ID are available to the therapist. In a concluding section, these will be considered and weighed from the perspective of the therapist wishing to enhance his or her capacity to enter the therapeutic relationship mindfully and skill-fully.

CULTIVATING MINDFULNESS IN RELATIONSHIP

A clear impression of ID practice will lay the foundation for considering how this new practice can enhance the quality of the therapist–client relationship.

A Snapshot of the Practice

In a group gathered for this practice, participants begin by calming down. They are invited to sit quietly and to become mindful of moment-to-moment bodily sensations. Then a meditation instruction or guideline is offered, along with a contemplation topic.

The guidelines provide needed support for awareness and letting go amid the challenges of relationship. The guidelines work together, synergistically, but are introduced one at a time in a careful sequence. They can be worked with separately, or used as reminders in daily life. Perhaps the guideline for this session is *Pause*. The facilitator might say, "I invite you to slow down, to find the present moment—here and now. Pause from habitual thoughts and reactions, Pause for a moment from being caught up in thinking; notice the body. What is the posture of the body now? What is the shape and form of the body? You might notice any sensations or tensions. Notice the sense of letting go of whatever you were doing or thinking. Pause."

After some individual meditation, participants are invited into pairs or larger groupings, and a contemplation topic is introduced. Perhaps this session's topic is aging. Participants might be told, "Each of us is subject to aging. Our bodies are changing; everyone we know is growing older: our parents and our children, our friends and our colleagues. How do you experience this? What does aging bring up for you right now? As you enter into dialogue, please remind yourself to Pause: to step out of reactions to your own or your meditation partner's story and become mindful of the body and of passing thoughts, and enter the relational moment fresh and awake. Pause into mindfulness as you explore the shared human experience of aging." When a bell is rung, the participants begin their dialogues. During the dialogue, the teacher or facilitator occasionally rings a bell to bring the meditators back to silent mindfulness and to help them further establish the meditative quality of their interactions. Participants are simultaneously cultivating the mindfulness of Pause and exploring an essential aspect of human experience.

The IMP and ID both involve a clearly defined role for the teacher or facilitator, who shares the guidelines, maintains the practice environment, and models the practice in how he or she relates to others. He or she works to create and sustain a safe container in which kindness, honesty, and commitment to practice can become the norm. In both settings, the teacher also rings the bell as a call to silence, offers short talks, and leads interludes of physical movement.

The classic lovingkindness meditation (outlined by Bien, Chapter 3, this volume; see also Salzberg, 1995) is used at the close of each IMP class period and at the close of ID sessions or days of practice. Like the contemplation topics and their consideration in dyads, lovingkindness meditation emphasizes acceptance and acknowledgment of kindness toward self and others, focusing the mind on the shared human experience. Participants begin to comprehend on a deeper level the fact that all beings share similar experiences, including pain, ease, and clear awareness. These insights support the capacity of lovingkindness practice to shift participants' perceptions of self and others.

Guidelines and Contemplations

The meditation instructions or *guidelines* and the use of *contemplations* form the core of the practice. ID (and its offshoot the IMP) are rooted in and shaped by the use of guidelines and contemplation topics. These guidelines are *Pause, Relax, Open, Trust Emergence, Listen Deeply,* and *Speak the Truth* (see Table 12.1).

Pause refers to a temporal pause from habitual thoughts and responses and an attitude of mindfulness toward experience in the present moment. In Pause, the practitioner becomes aware of himself or herself, and of the meditation partner(s), in a way that is less identified with emotional reactions. Reminding oneself to Pause, one steps out of the complex web of conditioning that arises in relationship and learns to create a space between what is heard, seen, or thought and one's responses, thereby developing the inner resources for stability and for making calm choices. Pause opens a doorway beyond relational habit patterns, through which one may step into nonclinging.

Relax invites the meditator to calm the body and mind, and to accept whatever thoughts and feelings are present in the moment. Relax points to an attitude of acceptance of difficult thoughts and emotions. Relax ripens into concentration and the unconditional acceptance of lovingkindness.

TABLE 12.1. Insight Dialogue Guidelines

Pause
  Temporal pause; step out of reaction and identification; mindfulness.

Relax
  Bodily calm; acceptance; tranquility; concentration; kindness.

Open
  Extension of mindfulness from internal to external; spaciousness; mutuality
  of practice.

Trust Emergence
  No agenda; flexibility; note impermanence of thoughts and feelings; "don't
  know" mind.

Listen Deeply
  Mindfulness while relating to others; receptivity; listen to meaning, emotions,
  and energetic presence.

Speak the Truth
  Mindfulness of speech; clarity of meaning, authenticity of emotion, and
  nonidentified presence; discernment of what to say amidst the universe
  of possibilities.

Open invites the participant to extend mindful and kind awareness beyond the boundaries of the mind and body to the external world, both environment and people. In Open one becomes aware of others with simple acceptance. Open is the spacious extension of meditation into the relational moment.

Trust Emergence means entering practice without any agenda; it engenders mental flexibility and appreciation for the impermanence and contingency of moment-to-moment experience. Trust Emergence points to "don't know mind" and to the vibrating quality of all phenomena. Open and Trust Emergence are explicit guidelines in ID but are not presented specifically in the IMP. The orientations they point to are embedded in the verbal instructions given during the IMP course, however.

Listen Deeply and *Speak the Truth* are a call to bring the authenticity and attunement of full presence into the moment of relationship. Listen Deeply begins with mindful and attuned listening. It ripens into full energetic presence and unhindered receptivity, to both words and other elements of interaction. When participants Listen Deeply to another, they are able to process information with less bias and to learn from what is spoken. A communication loop is created and maintained (Kramer, 1999, 2006).

Speak the Truth begins with the articulation of the simple truth of one's subjective experience. Discernment of what to speak and mindfulness while speaking are both elements of the guideline to Speak the Truth. Attunement to self and other is enhanced. Speak the Truth ripens into an acute sensitivity to the voice of the moment that "speaks through" the meditator.

Contemplations are the second central element of ID practice, and hence of the IMP also. The contemplations are topics of conversation drawn from Buddhist tradition, from other wisdom traditions, and from more modern framings of carefully observed human experience. They are selected to encourage a reevaluation of one's assumptions and behavior patterns and to foster deeper insight into the human condition. They also provide a present moment conversational basis for meditators as they use the guidelines to cultivate mindfulness, tranquility, adaptability, compassion, and the ability to respond authentically. The contemplations help guide the practice toward deeper recesses of experience, as revealed by mindfulness. They help the practitioner remain present with aspects of experience that he or she would just as soon ignore.

The contemplations are chosen to highlight significant elements of the shared human experience. They all have the implicit theme "What are the nature, dynamics, and qualities of my life?" Aging, disease, and death, lovingkindness and compassion, and the hungers for pleasure, recognition, and escape are all contemplation topics drawn from classical Buddhism. Traditional topics are used alongside topics like the roles assumed at work, at home, and in one's intimate relationships. Such topics are rarely discussed with others in an authentic yet nonreactive way. The act of discussing the contemplation material, the discovery of the universal nature of the stresses involved, and the meditation partner's calm acceptance all have a steadying effect on the participant.

The guidelines and contemplations work together synergistically. Self-knowledge deepens in relation to the contemplation themes as participants become more mindful and physiologically and emotionally more calm. The contemplations in turn foster engagement, which supports steadier mindfulness and calm. Trust builds among group members as each individual feels more at ease and realizes that individual responses to the contemplations are shared by others. Trust yields greater flexibility of mind states and deeper tranquility. Meditative mind states begin to arise in participants even while they are relationally engaged. Mindfulness, alertness, energetic presence, and investigation are balanced by kindness, tranquility, joy, concentration, and equanimity. Participants begin to recognize the causal relationship between grasping and suffering. With each moment of practice, they learn to choose ease and compassion over stress and self-identification.

The Emergence of ID and the IMP

Insight Dialogue rests on an understanding of the dharma that is very traditional, as well as a vision of interpersonal meditation and an interpersonal understanding of the dharma (Kramer, 2007). Its immediate roots include Gregory Kramer's early work with traditional Asian meditation teachers and study of Buddist psychology (the Abhidhamma), and an experiment in combining Bohmian dialogue and *vipassana* practice. With Terri O'Fallon, Kramer developed the first version of ID as an online practice, and together they produced a research methodology to study it and a joint PhD dissertation (Kramer & O'Fallon, 1997).

The practice evolved over the next several years as Kramer began teaching retreats and weekly groups. Many of ID's distinctive elements emerged in 2000 and 2001: breaking the group into subgroups, changing group sizes throughout the retreat, introducing explicit topics to the dialogue groups, including yoga to bring bodily ease, meditation in nature to encourage a gentle opening of awareness, and the occasional use of walking meditation in combination with dialogue. The introduction of contemplations drawn directly from the Buddha's teachings opened the door between ID and the other wisdom traditions—essential truths from any tradition are suitable as contemplation topics. The combination of mindfulness and calm concentration with contemplations is now the foundation of ID. At present (2007), ID has been taught to several thousand people in North America, Europe, Asia, and Australia; weekly groups engage the practice on three continents, and a group of senior teachers is being trained by Kramer.

The IMP dates from Kramer's invitation to Allie Rudolph and Yael Schweitzer to invite MBSR teachers to a special ID retreat sponsored by the Metta Foundation; the other participants were Katherine A. Bonus, Kaye H. Coker, Joan Fishman Hecht, and Florence Meleo-Meyer. After an intensive ID retreat taught by Kramer, this group began to consider curriculum development. Collaboration continued after the retreat, and the group fashioned a presentation of the basics of ID to fit the populations they expected to serve: mainstream, not explicitly Buddhist or especially committed to spiritual ideals, and motivated largely toward addressing daily problems and improving functioning. The Metta Foundation provided teacher training materials and authorized the use of the ID practice and the group's pilot offering in 2003.

Based on an informal evaluation in 2004–2005, the course was reduced from 8 weeks to 6 weeks and some of the busier aspects of the course, such as movement sessions, poetry, and music, were streamlined. Concerns for simplicity and accessibility also led to trimming down the practice guidelines from six to four. At present, the IMP explicitly presents only Pause, Relax, Listen Deeply, and Speak the Truth. (The remaining two guidelines, Open and Trust Emergence, were deemed too subtle for a short course and are no longer taught explicitly in the IMP; rather, they continue as implicit influences in the language used by the instructor.) Later revisions led to the current form of the course: an introductory class to review mindfulness practice, six class sessions, and one daylong retreat. At the time of writing (2007), the IMP has been offered for 4 years in pilot projects at several university medical centers and in private therapy practice.

The Logic of Interpersonal Meditation

All of these forms—ID retreats, weekly groups, online meditation, the IMP, and other forms under development—share in the logic of interpersonal meditation: its ability to foster attitudes and responses that transfer readily into other relationships. This logic also includes the powerful dynamics of mutuality. When people meditate together and one becomes distracted or overly identified with his or her emotions, others can supply the reminder—through words or behavior—to return to mindfulness, to relax and accept present experience. A feedback loop is created, reinforcing energy and clarity and opening new understanding. Mutuality also supports the natural tendency of the open and accepting mind toward lovingkindness and compassion. Thus interpersonal meditation reveals the intersubjective nature of experience—the shared human experience in the moment it is lived.

THERAPEUTIC STANCES AND SKILLS SUPPORTED BY ID

Mindfulness can be integrated into therapeutic work in a variety of ways. Germer (2005) divides these into three groups, all of which are compatible with ID. The ID guidelines point to specific skills that can be immediately useful for persons receiving psychotherapy. Elements of the practice, such as the use of the guideline Pause, can be taught to the client—in Germer's terminology, this would be Mindfulness-Based Psychotherapy. For example, Kim and Kramer (2002) taught the ID guidelines to people with social anxiety disorders, with promising results. ID's theoretical frames of reference can also inform therapy, with or without any explicit teaching: this would be Mindfulness-Informed Psychotherapy. We consider this option, albeit briefly and with reference to ID's context in Buddhism, in the next section of this chapter.

The focus of this section, however, is on the therapist's practice of interpersonal mindfulness as it enhances and supports the therapist–client relationship.[1] In Germer's terminology, we will be exploring ID's contribution to Mindfulness-Oriented Psychotherapy. ID in all its forms, including the IMP, can support therapists in their relationships with clients. A number of aspects of the therapeutic relationship are treated here, grouped under the headings of therapist self-awareness and acceptance, the capacity to be present to and accepting of the client, and the fruits of practice in exploring present moment experience in relationship. The ID guidelines have significant depths that unfold only with time and practice. In intensive practice, the guidelines and the meditative skills they point to are practiced repeatedly; in longer retreats, they often yield exceptional clarity and stillness. Mindfulness, tranquility, energy, and inquiry gradually become a natural mode of being in relationship.

Support for Therapist Self-Awareness and Acceptance

An important group of factors in the therapist–client relationship can be considered as dimensions of therapist self-awareness and self-acceptance. These include acceptance of dysphoric experiences during the therapy session, such as not knowing what is going on, not knowing what to do, countertransference phenomena, and needs and pressures that emerge into consciousness from the therapist's life situation.

Pause at its most literal level—pausing before speaking—provides an interruption of any tendency the therapist may have to respond automatically. Not knowing what to do or say can be experienced as dysphoric, dangerous. The Pause enables the therapist to recognize his or her self-identification with being the knowing one, the competent helper who must have and provide answers. As the gesture of non-identification, Pause also allows the therapist to step back from identification with negative feelings and so prevent their escalation. Without identification with these roles, there is the possibility of meeting the client with what Shunryu Suzuki (1973) called "beginner's mind." Trust Emergence, in particular, can extend this: trusting what emerges frees the therapist from having an agenda, from having to accomplish something. Speak the Truth, in combination with these qualities, fosters patience and discernment, freeing the therapist to accept silences and to wait for the emergence of what is relevant in this moment.

Countertransference reactions in particular may be seen by therapists as dangerous, confusing, embarrassing, or inadmissible. The guidelines Pause and Relax help the therapist recognize, accept, and respond effectively to his or her own reactivity and/or countertransference. Practicing Pause supports the therapist's mindful awareness of his or her reactions and emotions, and allows them to be examined rather than defended against. In the therapeutic moment, Pause introduces a buffer between reaction and action or expression. When Pause uncovers difficult matters, it needs the support of Relax. The initial, literal Relaxing matures into deep acceptance and compassion. Over time, meeting troublesome inner phenomena with stillness means that they are not fed; their energy begins to drain out of them.

Therapists are often challenged to be aware of how personal needs affect the therapeutic relationship. Home and work roles can easily intertwine, and one may impinge upon the other. Emotional reactions and personal stories may interfere with the therapist's ability to be attentive. ID offers the calm acceptance of the guideline Relax; with the guidelines Pause and Trust Emergence, the therapist can increase his or her awareness of the flow, intensity, and impermanence of inner emotional and thought formations, especially as they arise in dialogue with another. Mindful awareness of reactive judgments as they arise does not imply passivity, but allows flexibility and choice of actions. The therapist's personal practice of mindfulness and compassion becomes a valuable resource and model for clients struggling in their relationships. Clear, unattached awareness of these emotions and thoughts supports the therapist in showing up as a whole person—the foundation of being fully and effectively present to another.

Presence to the Client, Empathy

The stance of unconditional presence is, in turn, known to assist the healing process (Welwood, 1992). Such unconditional presence is manifested as the presence of the whole person, present moment empathy, and the therapist's genuine interest and close attention.

The guideline Open is the primary reminder to the practitioner to extend meditative awareness from the personal to the interpersonal. When applied to the therapeutic relationship, Open invites the therapist to notice the "between" of relationship. The sense of an isolated self and separate other give way to an I–Thou relationship, as experienced in ID practice. The mindfulness and calm concentration of meditation are repurposed for relationship and open the way for the emergence of present moment empathy.

Empathy with the client in the present moment is especially supported by the guidelines Relax and Open. These two motions powerfully support the stances Buddhism knows as the *brahmaviharas* or "divine abidings"—lovingkindness, compassion, joy, and equanimity. These may be considered as aspects of the awareness, understanding, and sensitivity referred to as empathy. They are the fruits of mental training, not simply emotional states (as Thomas Bien notes in Chapter 3), and can be cultivated by the therapist in an especially effective way in ID.

Buddhist psychology considers aversion as a kind of tension or stress. As the gesture of Relax—the letting go of tension—ripens, a state of nonaversion necessarily takes its place. Nonaversion is the basis of these four qualities; they arise naturally and spontaneously in the absence of aversion. Lovingkindness, compassion, and sympathetic joy become strong when Relax is opened outward to the other. Open fosters awareness of and responsiveness to the other's condition and extends meditative awareness into the "between" of relationship. Equanimity is also strongly evoked by Trust Emergence and develops the balance needed to remain available and responsive in a changing or challenging situation.

Equanimity, especially as developed relationally through Relax and Trust Emergence, is an invaluable resource in the difficult moments of therapy. Without the balance provided by this combination of Relax, Open, and Trust Emergence, it is difficult to remain available and responsive to a client's pain, anger, confusion, or blame without being pulled off balance. In the face of ambiguity, silence, and strong affect, Relax and Trust Emergence—and their fruits of compassion and equanimity—allow genuine openness for the client to coexist with the self-awareness required to self-regulate naturally. When Relax has been practiced in the relational context of interpersonal meditation, it becomes a strong support for recognizing tension and choosing ease. It engenders deep acceptance of self and other.

The Fruits of Practice in Interpersonal Meditation

Especially when the guidelines are practiced with precision and with the support of other meditators, ID presents an unparalleled opportunity to experience and explore unbinding in relationship. As stress, fear, distraction, and longing are revealed, they can be dropped; they no longer block the channel; mutuality emerges naturally.

The therapist practicing ID also gains experience in how it is to be in relationship with another who is also cultivating these qualities, enjoying the unbinding of another and thereby gaining direct personal experience of therapeutic change and transformation. Deep listening takes on an entirely new dimension. Speaking the truth is understood as arising from the body, from the deeper recesses of the heart-mind, and from emptiness. Relational wisdom—the intersubjective presence that is essential for good therapy—is experienced in the body, and in the felt sense of the moment, with the precision of refined mindfulness.

In ID, these qualities are developed and explored while in relationship with others.

RESOURCES IN BUDDHISM FOR SUPPORTING THE THERAPEUTIC RELATIONSHIP

The theoretical frame of therapy can also be informed by ID—an instance of Germer's category, Mindfulness-Informed Psychotherapy (2005). Since ID is based in and indeed incorporates Buddhism's frame of reference, psychological insights, and goals, this is an especially rich possibility. The Buddhist orientations of the practice are clearly defined, and certain qualities of psychological growth are named. These orientations and qualities underlie the IMP also, but are not named or taught as explicitly there.

Buddhism as a Psychology

Western observers, perhaps beginning with William James (1902/1982), have identified Buddhism as primarily a school of psychology; James (prematurely) remarked, "This is the psychology everybody will be studying twenty-five years from now" (Scott, 2000). While without religious overtones, ID is firmly embedded in the psychological understandings and practices of Buddhism. ID teachers refer directly to the Buddha's teachings, making use of the richness and precision of Buddhist psychological concepts and terminology. ID is explicitly guided by Buddhism's long established ethical and pedagogical system and its rich epistemology.

Buddhism's Contexts for Human Transformation

The Four Noble Truths of Buddhism address human suffering at its
root. They are supported by a body of observations and practices that
have been tested for millennia. Buddhism's diagnosis is that suffering is
self-elaborated by means of hunger in its various forms (which include
the cravings for pleasure, for recognition, and for escape). Buddhism's
prescription, the Eightfold Path, is a multimodal, synergistic approach.
Mindfulness is only one part of this prescription—or rather, Right
Mindfulness is: skillful mindfulness, mindfulness that tends toward the
lessening of suffering. Mindfulness *can* take unskilled, unhelpful forms—
awareness oriented toward fixing or enhancing the self, or a means of
escape from life's realities. As one element of the Eightfold Path, the
broad attentiveness to the present moment called Mindfulness takes its
place as a quality of attention beside the strong natural focus of the calm
mind, Right Concentration. The energetic application of both Mindfulness and Concentration, when directed toward the release of unwholesome mental states and behaviors and the cultivation of wholesome
ones, is called Right Effort.

Even these attentional qualities—Right Effort, Mindfulness, and
Concentration—are only part of the prescribed regimen. The full prescription also includes a moral triad: Right Speech, Right Action, and
Right Lifestyle. These checkpoints do not exist to promote conformity
to culturally or religiously sanctioned conventions, but because their
neglect has been proven to increase suffering and to negate the benefits
of the attentional qualities of Right Effort, Right Mindfulness, and Right
Calm Concentration. Neglecting ethical behavior clouds the mind. It
can lead to actions that hurt others, which further cloud the mind.
Mind and behavior always affect each other; it is impossible to cultivate
goodness in one without the other. "Right" in this context means
"effective"—it refers to the speech, action, and lifestyle qualities that
have been shown empirically to reduce self-caused and self-elaborated
suffering. An approach to life options that appeals to empirically ob-
servable consequences, rather than to cultural or religious conventions
which may not be shared, is eminently adapted as a frame of reference
for therapeutic work.

These factors are prefaced, in the Eightfold Path, by the need for
understanding of cause and effect in one's mental and emotional life—
Right View—and by a commitment to using that understanding to re-
orient one's life and actions towards relinquishment and kindness—
Right Intention. Right View also encompasses a clear understanding of

the cause of suffering and the remarkable human potential to end this suffering. Without an understanding of how suffering is caused and elaborated, and the will to take hold of the laws of psychological causality, the development of attention—or any of the other factors—becomes a trivial nicety. They work together, not in isolation, and ID is intended to be part of this process.

Mindfulness plays a role in another part of Buddhism's psychology. It is one element in a series of qualities that each lead to the next, and that together support the clear perception of reality. These qualities are Mindfulness, Inquiry, Energy, Joy, Tranquility, Concentration, and Equanimity. The abstraction of mindfulness from these contexts and its application in the West have sometimes been marked by a broadening of the word's meaning to encompass several of these qualities—for example, inquiry and tranquility; both clarity and precision are lost in the process. When the natural sequence of this list, in which each quality is the ground of the next, is understood, there is more for the practitioner—or the therapist—to work with. ID, while radical in its *direct* application of the dharma to interpersonal relationships, is traditional and explicit in its endeavor to cultivate this wider panoply of mental qualities.

The ancient and sophisticated psychology that is Buddhism also differs in its goal from the young and evolving Western psychologies. The Western psychologies typically aim at the diminishment of suffering by a mixed bouquet of approaches: gaining the social skills to get one's needs met more effectively, adjusting one's wants to the surrounding context of what is accepted and possible, resolving buried past conflicts of many kinds, integration of the self. Western psychologies have articulated their goals in diverse ways also, based on their different assessments of the nature of the human being. These young disciplines are in a stage of yeasty ferment, offering much that is useful and containing fresh insights and wisdom. They are also beginning to draw a great deal directly from Buddhist teachings. But as a group they are ambiguous in their analysis of human nature and the root cause(s) of suffering, and they change with the fashions of the passing decades.

The Buddha's psychology aims bluntly at the end of suffering: its cessation. It proposes to reach that end by the complete relinquishment of the cause of suffering, *hunger* or *craving* in the specific, technical sense assigned to these terms. The cessation of craving, in turn, is inextricably linked with the eradication of ignorance about the constructed, impersonal nature of the self, as Fulton discusses in Chapter 4 of this volume. Buddhism's prescription also results in the lessening of suffering along the way to this startling goal of suffering's abolition—but in contrast to Western psychologies, it pursues this lessening from the perspective of a single coherent analysis of suffering's cause. The "methodology" underlying its millennia of evaluative efforts is simple: is a given practice or program effective in moving people along the path of relinquishment of the root cause of suffering, as evidenced in the actual lessening of suffering?

Buddhism's empirical approach has produced other refinements of understanding that support the lessening of suffering. The cultivation of specific qualities of mind such as lovingkindness and compassion, for example, has evolved both practical approaches of great refinement and valuable working definitions of those qualities. In a similar way, ID draws from and offers as part of its practice such penetrating insights of Buddhist psychology as dependent origination (*Paticca-samuppada Sutta* [SN 12.1]), the aggregates of clinging (*Nakulapi Sutta* [SN 22.1]), and the wholesome and unwholesome roots of thought (*Sammaditthi Sutta* [MN 9.4-7]). Taken together, this rich blend of theory and practice help ensure ID's continued development in scope and depth.

Because ID draws explicitly from the Buddha's teachings, certain orientations of the practice are clearly defined, and certain qualities of psychological growth are named. The hungers for pleasure, for narcissistic satisfaction, and for escape (escape often manifests interpersonally as a fear of intimacy) are understood as foundational, so one learns to recognize and release them rather than to satisfy them more efficiently. This focus on relinquishment is explicit and its practice is embedded in how ID is taught. The practice of relinquishment takes place within a moral context, and an important part of this process is represented by the system of *dana*, or generosity. This system, still young in the West, insists that the teaching be offered freely: teachers are not paid for their teachings, which are considered priceless. Rather, meditators are encouraged to engage in the practice of generosity: they offer support to the teachers as they are personally moved to do so, with the hope that this will help keep the teachings available, allowing others to benefit as they have done. Because ID is offered on this *dana* basis, it is effectively lifted from the challenges and distortions inherent in commercial enterprises and in the development of a professional practice.

When therapists not only gain some measure of personal transformation in ID but also understand the dynamics of transformation as laid out in Buddhist psychology, they have a schema for discerning and guiding transformation in their clients as well.

INTERPERSONAL MEDITATION
TRAINING OPTIONS FOR THERAPISTS

Considered as an approach to developing therapeutic presence, ID is one that uses the same methods in training as in the actual work (see Gehart & McCollum, Chapter 11, this volume). Germer (2005) indicates that the extent to which mindfulness is to be implemented in psychotherapy may influence the degree of training and practice needed. The developers of Mindfulness-Based Cognitive Therapy (MBCT) conclude that "after seeing for ourselves the difference between using MBCT with and without personal experience of using mindfulness practice, it is unwise for instructors to embark on teaching this material before they have extensive personal experience with its use" (Segal, Williams, & Teasdale, 2002, p. 84). We concur that it is imperative for the therapist wishing to benefit from ID to gain as much personal experience with the practice as possible.

Open Enrollment Options

The therapist or other helping professional can enter and benefit from ID practice through any of its manifestations. An initial "taste" of the practice could be had by participating as a student in an IMP class, participating in a weekly group, or attending one of the shorter ID retreats. These are avenues that a therapist might pursue for the enrichment of his or her practice but might also recommend to a client. Meditators enter into ID in the same way; it should be noted that the peer-to-peer nature of the dialogues can pose some initial challenge to therapists new to it.

The IMP provides a very solid, if basic, introduction to the practice. In comparison to the other ID formats, connections with Western psychology, while not presented explicitly in the IMP, may be more readily gleaned by a therapist–participant. On the other hand, there will be less of the conceptual framework of Buddhist psychology available for informing and guiding therapeutic practice.

Weekly ID groups, led by a facilitator, are also an option. Weekly groups progress through a programmed 8-week introduction to ID and then continue meeting and practicing together, revisiting the practice guidelines and exploring new contemplations. The material covered in the introductory sequence is roughly similar to that of the IMP, although the guidelines Open and Trust Emergence are fully included. ID facilitators are not required to be as thoroughly trained as IMP teachers.

The chief advantages to weekly groups are the integration of practice with everyday life (in contrast to retreat formats) and the opportunity to continue working on interpersonal meditation as a group over the following months or even years (in contrast to the IMP).

ID retreats come in a variety of durations, from one day to more than a week. Retreats of just a few days can provide a solid, if basic, introduction to the practice. ID retreats take a form similar to insight meditation retreats: there are periods of silent sitting meditation and of interpersonal ID meditation; there are periods for walking meditation or rest. Meals are taken in silence, and participants refrain from interactions apart from the ID sessions. The focus is on the practice.

Greater depth can be had by attending longer ID retreats. While ID can be beneficial in any of its forms, it reaches its fullest development in the setting of a longer retreat. In retreat, the qualities pointed to by the guidelines ripen over the longer course of intensive practice. Hence, retreatants are able to experience these qualities to an exceptional degree. Retreat practice opens up the possibility of deep insight in the midst of interpersonal contact. A qualitatively deeper experience of lovingkindness and compassion and a radical release of one's sense of self and other are not uncommon experiences in these longer retreats.

Options with Restricted Enrollment

Some other opportunities exist that are restricted in several different ways.

Some ID retreats are offered specifically for therapists. These typically include contemplation themes drawn from the practice of therapy and greater attention to the psychological framework supplied by Buddhism. Most of these are longer retreats.

For one specific subgroup of therapists only—those who have completed the full course of training offered for MBSR teachers by the Center for Mindfulness at the University of Massachusetts Medical School—there is the option to train to teach the IMP. In the course of the prerequisite MBSR training, they will have participated in silent *vipassana* retreats, developed and maintained a regular meditation practice, and received in-depth training in the theory and curriculum associated with MBSR. It is also expected that IMP teachers will have group process skills and some familiarity with psychotherapeutic approaches.

In the IMP training itself, prospective teachers participate in multiple ID retreats, some of them paired with detailed teacher training.

These retreats provide firsthand experience of the guidelines and contemplations. They also offer direct experience of in-depth practice and the personal transformation it enables, thus enhancing the prospective teachers' capacities for nonreactive, relational presence. The training sessions help IMP teachers to understand the many layers of instruction inherent in the six simple guidelines, to gain an overview of the theory behind ID and the IMP, and to grow through the unique interpersonal dynamics actuated in the practice. It is expected that IMP teachers will continue their traditional (silent) meditation practice, and that they will pursue further ID training.

Two other training opportunities exist, but they are linked with formats that can only be offered free of charge, in accordance with the tradition of *dana* (generosity). Because of this, they are not suitable for therapists wishing only or primarily to improve their professional practice—though therapists are by no means barred from them. The first is the facilitation of a weekly ID group. Facilitators are required to have an established meditation practice and a specified level of experience with ID; they receive ongoing support and training from the Metta Foundation as they facilitate the weekly group. The second option is training as an ID teacher. ID teacher trainees work as apprentices co-teaching with Gregory Kramer, at first teaching only short nonresidential retreats on their own. They attend teachers' meetings, participate in teleconferences, and work in pairs or triads. Although it uses new technologies, this training remains in many respects an apprenticeship training modeled after traditional Asian teacher training relationships.

Information on various trainings and retreats can be found at *www.metta.org* and (for the IMP) *www.umassmed.edu/cfm*.

CONCLUSION

Mindfulness is an innate human capacity, and ID is about being human in a wise and compassionate way. ID is revolutionary in cultivating mindfulness and associated qualities directly in relationship, thus easing their transfer into other relationships. It can be understood as a means of personal transformation or as a resource for therapist training. In addition, the deeper framework of Buddhist psychology undergirding ID (and the IMP) offers breathtaking psychological insights that can guide therapeutic practice for therapists so inclined. ID is the most direct approach we know to bringing mindfulness into relationship. From the perspective of therapist training or continuing education, ID's potential stems from its fostering of mindfulness in the place where the greatest difference can be made: in relationship.

NOTE

1. We wish to thank Sharon Beckman-Brindley for generously sharing her insights on the role of the guidelines in supporting the therapeutic relationship.

REFERENCES

Germer, C. K. (2005). Teaching mindfulness in therapy. In C. K. Germer, R. D. Siegel, & P. R. Fulton (Eds.), *Mindfulness and psychotherapy* (pp. 55–72). New York: Guilford Press.

James, W. (1982). *Varieties of religious experience.* New York: Viking Penguin. (Original work published 1902)

Kim, J., & Kramer, G. (2002). Insight Dialogue meditation with anxiety problems. *Gestalt!*, 6(1). Available at *www.g-gej.org/6-1/insightdialogue.html.*

Kramer, G. (1999). *Meditating together, speaking from silence: The practice of Insight Dialogue.* Portland, OR: Metta Foundation.

Kramer, G. (2006). Deep listening: An interview with Gregory Kramer. *Insight Journal, 26,* 4–8.

Kramer, G. (2007). *Insight Dialogue: The interpersonal path to freedom.* Boston: Shambhala.

Kramer, G., & O'Fallon, T. (1997). *Insight dialogue and insight dialogic inquiry.* Unpublished doctoral dissertation, California Institute of Integral Studies, San Francisco.

Nakulapita sutta (SN 22.1).

Paticca-samuppada sutta (SN 12.1).

Salzberg, S. (1995). *Lovingkindness: The revolutionary art of happiness.* Boston: Shambhala.

Sammaditthi sutta (MN 9.4-7).

Scott, D. (2000). William James and Buddhism: American pragmatism and the Orient. *Religion, 30,* 335.

Segal, Z. V., Williams, J. M. G., & Teasdale, J. D. (2002). *Mindfulness-based cognitive therapy for depression: A new approach to preventing relapse.* New York: Guilford Press.

Suzuki, S. (1973). *Zen mind, beginner's mind.* Trumble, CT: Weatherhill.

Welwood, J. (1992). The healing power of unconditional presence. In J. Welwood (Ed.), *Ordinary magic: Everyday life as spiritual path* (pp. 159–170). Boston: Shambhala.

13 Mindful Listening for Better Outcomes

REBECCA SHAFIR

As I walk down to the waiting room to greet Abby, my next patient, I look forward to hearing the latest accounts of this restless soul. So
far, she is making progress in communicating more effectively with her family, but there are still some sticking points to work through. I say a prayer to
help me remember to hear what she is trying to tell me. I hope that by being
heard, she will be able to better understand herself. I set my mind to forget
my agenda for the next hour.

With a few more steps to go, I wonder how Freud, Reik, Jung, and all
the other great psychoanalysts would hear Abby today. How would they
have managed long hours of listening if they had been taxed by the demands
of multitasking, a crowded schedule, and the Internet's tempting torrent of
information? Spared the vagaries of managed care paperwork, the cell
phone vibrating in their pocket, and the laptop blinking in the corner, I suspect they were able to stay vigilant for hours, picking up the subtlest of
subtlties. Perhaps, back then, their offices were more like dens: noiseless,
cozy, and devoid of interruptions. I also suspect that since external distractions were fewer in those days, a clinician's internal distractions (worry,
time stresses, feelings of being overwhelmed, etc.) may have been less. Were
their minds more at ease? Did they have more "mental space" available for
their patients? I envy how much easier it might have been to listen deeply
back then. I wonder what I would have heard then that, with all good intentions, I don't hear now.

In light of this modern-day dilemma, might today's clinicians compensate for these external distractions by finding ways to enhance their relationships with their patients by a more conscious way of listening? And with regular mindfulness practice, could clinicians help their patients, burdened too with a host of internal distractions, learn to listen better to others?

I am a speech–language pathologist and a neurotherapist. Psychologists and psychiatrists refer patients to me who need to improve their cognitive and communication skills. My outcomes rely heavily upon the quality of my listening skills and my ability to teach these skills to patients. Listening is part of the healing process; it is what a therapist does best and what patients depend on, since they can not always hear themselves.

My purpose in writing this chapter is to offer some practical guidelines for refining a clinician's listening ability, which will, in turn, enhance his or her relationships with patients, thus leading to more successful outcomes. Many patients present with significant interpersonal communication challenges stemming from various mental conditions and disorders. For a clinical relationship to be truly *therapeutic,* patients need to walk away with more than just a decrease in symptoms. They need to experience, in the context of a meaningful relationship, an understanding of what healthy communication is all about.

Whether one chooses to share these skills indirectly by example or offer a skill-based therapy approach, it is necessary for a clinician to examine his or her own foundation for listening. The most authentic and reliable approach to listening has its source in mindfulness. Mindful listening is not so much a skill or a method as it is an *attitude,* or a *state of mind.* It combines concentration and focus with curiosity and caring.

Clinicians who interact with patients from a mindful listening perspective do so with the intent of *partnering* with their patients. Any successful partnership requires trust between parties. Trust is a key element of a therapeutic relationship; it is an element that, if it develops, does so over time. Trust embodies many of the essentials of mindfulness as it has been described in earlier chapters. Creating trust within a therapeutic relationship means being *aware* of the needs of patients, *attentive* and responsive to those needs, and *accepting* and *present in the moment* for them. Patients need to know that a therapist understands and accept them; only then can patients feel that they can rely on his or her advice. Mindful listening helps therapists understand their patients well beyond the surface layer of words, test results, and historical accounts. Mindful listening fosters trust within a therapeutic relationship. Patients learn to trust that their clinician will accept them unconditionally for their strengths and their shortcomings. In a trusting therapeutic relationship, unlike most of their other, nonclinical relationships, the barriers of status, prejudice, or unrealistic expectations are less formidable.

As trust grows, patients begin to feel comfortable entertaining other points of view and become more open to the *possibility* of change. They become more receptive to and compliant with suggestions that stretch beyond their comfort zone. A healthy sense of trust inspires honest dialogue between patient and clinician; it becomes easier to voice differences of opinion. These quality exchanges help guide the clinician in planning and in responding to the patients needs. A patient's attendance in therapy becomes more consistent as a function of the positive, steady growth that is taking place. It is implicitly understood in any trusting relationship that mistakes can happen on both sides; but, if well intentioned, mistakes can be forgiven and accepted as part of the learning process.

Another positive therapeutic result of this partnership approach is that when trust is established in a clinical relationship, it helps patients develop an inner trust of themselves. Patients become more self-confident and independent in "right" decision making. The true litmus test of the therapeutic effectiveness of the clinical relationship is how well patients are able to apply these same lessons to their relationships *outside therapy*. Patients want more than just a sounding board. They seek out the kind of therapeutic assistance that will empower and enable them to navigate the unsteady seas of interpersonal relationships.

WHY NOT LISTENING 101?

My interest in listening resulted from teaching a listening course to managers at my hospital. The risk management department supplied me with documents that outlined the costly consequences of poor listening for patient care and the health care system. In contrast with these poor results, successful outcomes (not necessarily *cures*) reportedly were the result of a positive connection between patients and their health care provider (HCP)—so much so, that even if something went wrong in treatment, these patients were less likely to consider litigation. There wasn't much research that could demonstrate this connection, much less how to teach it. Therefore, some fieldwork in the form of chart reviews and both patient and HCP interviews was needed to reveal the core characteristics of the therapeutic relationships that led to positive outcomes. Such outcomes might include not only a cure for patient symptoms, but also a reduced need for medications, a healthier quality of life, increased assertiveness, and greater ability to handle stress.

Reflecting upon their experiences, most of these patients claimed that the clinicians who facilitated the greatest gains reframed the meaning of their disorder by:

- Listening to them and offering an explanation for the problem that made sense.
- Using a strengths-based approach that fostered greater self-acceptance.
- Offering practical strategies for dealing with difficult people and situations.

From this exploration came the call for mindful listening. Now I was determined to identify mindful listeners, learn from them, and figure out ways to teach what they do to others.

To a greater or lesser or extent, many clinicians have experienced the capacity for mindful listening, a little like those great psychotherapists who lived in a quieter time and place. In those moments they were able to shut out internal and external distractions. Such moments, which with practice can be extended, are similar to the calm, egoless, present-tense state that meditators experience. In those moments when clinicians forgot themselves and allowed their patients' agendas to take center stage, they entered into a deeper level of awareness and communication. It is in a state of mindfulness that the therapist is best able to capture the microfacial expressions, an inflection in the voice, the duration of a pause, a swallowing in the throat, or a slight movement of the body that gives richness and depth to the spoken words. Generous, attentive silence gives them the time and assurance to organize their thoughts and get to the depth of their concerns. When the therapist can listen this way, he or she can feel light despite a heavy schedule.

Listening is so basic to one's success with learning and relationships, and so threatened by this age of distraction, it is surprising that it is not taught early on. Training children to listen mindfully might directly improve grades and could curb schoolyard violence. Teaching parents how to listen to their children helps create good models and healthier connections at home. Premarital training in listening could conceivably lower the divorce rate. Infusing mindful listening into therapy sessions creates ripple effects. Once patients are heard mindfully and given the tools to listen mindfully themselves, they can directly improve relationships with family, friends, and coworkers. Family members will comment on positive changes in their loved ones' ability to talk through touchy subjects, interrupt less, and remember more of what they heard. These friends and family, in turn, tend to be, over time, a bit more patient and thoughtful with their own friends and co-workers.

Corporations know the benefits from listening to customers effectively. However, resources to provide effective listening training are feeble at best. In researching my book *The Zen of Listening* (2003), I visited corporations that taught listening as a part of their customer service training. The vast majority taught what I call "act-like-you're listening" techniques packaged in a three-, five-, or 10-step plan. Participants were taught to mirror the posture of the speaker, lean in, fix their gaze, and nod themselves senseless as the speaker spoke. Little or no attention was paid to improving concentration, which is often where listeners fall short. Listeners who are focused on techniques and maneuvers will miss a great deal of what is said and left unsaid. Mindful listeners maintain good eye contact and nod every so often, but these are reflexive responses to authentic connection. They are not planned in advance, and there is no intent to trick the speaker into *believing* they are truly being heard.

Most clinicians I interviewed had developed a rich ability to connect with their patients in their internships and residencies. However, over time, as many can attest, distractions and time constraints combine with the neediness of patients to diminish their capacity to listen freshly every time.

WHAT IS A MINDFUL LISTENER?

When I speak to groups of clinicians on the subject of mindful listening, I always ask for a show of hands of those who can recall when they were heard *wholeheartedly* even once in their lives. Without fail, sadly, only a few hands surface. Interestingly, these students will say it was a grandparent or a therapist who heard them in this way. When I explored these recollections with the "mindfully heard minority" they reported that that special listener generally demonstrated four qualities that made conversation with them memorable and often life changing. These listeners were able to:

1. *Sustain their attention* over time,
2. Hear and see the *whole message*,
3. Make the speaker feel *valued and respected*, and
4. Listen to *themselves.*

These characteristics define the essence of the *mindful listener.*

Meditation has long been known as a natural way of improving concentration. As an undergraduate in college I sought out transcendental meditation to help me deal with a demanding course load, opera school, and two part-time jobs. Over the years I explored various forms of meditation, including both concentration and mindfulness techniques. For the purpose of improving one's listening skills, both methods have their strengths and drawbacks. *Concentration* is about focusing on one thing at a time. In *concentration meditation* one may sit very still and focus on repeating a mantra, on the breath, or on a candle's flame. This kind of concentration practice helps one build mental power and focus for cultivation of the ability to stay calm in the present moment. *Mindfulness,* however, is about openness to whatever thought arises in the present moment; there is no attachment to any one thing or sensation. Mindfulness practice allows one to experience the full range of an activity. Thich Nhat Hanh, in his book *The Miracle of Mindfulness* (1987) gives the example of "washing the dishes to wash the dishes." While washing the dishes we simultaneously reflect upon the miracle of the process, its purpose, the touch and feel, and so forth. We are engaged in the present tense throughout the activity, conscious of the blending of our thoughts and actions. Practicing concentration makes it easier to stay focused, creating stability of mind. But a single focused practice has a more closed and less receptive quality than mindfulness practice. To focus on only one thing may lead a listener to miss what someone is expressing physically or emotionally. Mindfulness practice, however, is about opening and receiving rather than pushing away what we dislike, giving one's awareness a more investigative, curious flavor. However, it's easier to lose one's focus with mindfulness practice, and it can interfere with cultivating the stillness that leads to greater insight. Sensation-based *vipassana* (Glickman, 2002) is preferred by many of my patients and students, as it combines the best elements of both concentration and mindfulness practice. Body scanning and awareness of the full range of our emotions in the present moment train us to stay engaged in the listening process. As the Buddha taught, both concentration and awareness must be developed to achieve insight (Glickman, 2002).

Many of my patients claim that even with short periods of regular, daily meditation practice they are more inclined to notice when a distraction takes over. They notice their digressions and snap back into the present tense more quickly. Ideally, regular meditation practice of 20 minutes twice a day may help one achieve these results in a shorter period of time.

   Many of my students have reported mindful walking to be a doable and enjoyable approach. The fact that walking is something we do anyway (to the waiting room, the bathroom, our car, the staff room, etc.) makes it easier to cultivate the habit of pairing the act of walking with a quiet mind. I often start therapy sessions with a mindful walking session outdoors, weather permitting. There is no pressure for patients to look at me, they can look straight ahead and walk and listen to my cues. They think it as an exercise taught by a personal trainer.

   During this time, I don't bring up any difficult questions or give advice. We only walk and breathe for about 15–20 minutes. Clinicians can learn a great deal about their patients in this short period of time and vice versa. Some giggle nervously, others want to talk incessantly or complain about something or someone. The therapist gets to see how long it takes some persons to settle down after getting lost or being unable to find a parking place. Patients experience how the therapist listens nonjudgmentally and gently refocuses their attention on walking and the breath. After a few minutes they quiet down, realizing that all that fuss is a waste of energy. Silently counting the breath, inhaling on two steps and exhaling on four or five steps, is unobtrusive and centering. For those who prefer a more active form of meditation, *qi gong* and tai chi produce similar effects. Many patients who expected to start off sitting in my office, face to face with my clipboard, will remark upon this refreshing way to clear their mind of the "extranium" and make the most out of the session.

   I enjoy seeing patients warming up in the parking lot prior to their sessions. At home they start to include brief walks in their daily regimen to establish clarity for the day. They become aware of the "monkey in the brain" that jumps from one idea to another without restraint. These first steps are very helpful for patients with ADD/ADHD (attention-deficit disorder/attention-deficit/hyperactivity disorder), or attention-deficit traits, a term coined by Edward Hallowell (Hallowell & Ratey, 1994), who exhibit impulsivity, lack of focus, and thought organization problems that affect their communication effectiveness.

   We often close a session with 5 minutes of sitting meditation. This helps set the mind on a positive course to follow through on the plan we established. Patients with ADD/ADHD are encouraged by studies done by such researchers as Andrew Newberg and Eugene d'Aquili (2001) of the University of Pennsylvania. They used single-photon-emission computed tomography images of the brains of skilled meditators to show increased activity in the prefrontal cortex, the seat of attention.

   Meditation seems to condition the brain to listen. Interviews with seasoned meditators revealed that regular practice *predisposes* the body and the mind to listen in many ways. It helps us become comfortable with silence. It deautomatizes and dampens our response to "hot buttons," allowing more space and thoughtfulness between what the speaker says and our reaction to it. Meditation helps one move out from a rigid in-turned frame of reference to a more flexible interrelatedness. As Herbert Benson reported in his groundbreaking book *The Relaxation Response* (1975), meditation calms our heart rate and lowers our blood pressure even during stressful conversations. While sitting with our eyes closed we become more aware of the noise in our brains, and the layers of barriers that pop up in the midst of a conversation—past experiences, worries about the future, negative self-talk, judgment of our conversational partner, sex, and so on. With regular meditation practice, we learn to smile at these digressions, let them pass, and get back to the business of understanding the person speaking.

LISTENING TO THE NONVERBAL MESSAGE

Meditation ripens one's capacity to take in the *whole message*—not just the words, but the gestures, the facial expressions, the tone of voice, and the meaningful pauses. When we are able to quiet our minds, we are better able to capture more of the heart of the message. Albert Mehrabian (1972), a researcher in nonverbal communication, found that 7% of the meaning of an utterance is in the words that are spoken, 38% of meaning is paralinguistic (the way that the words are said), and 55% of meaning is in facial expression. Theodor Reik's most famous book, *Listening with the Third Ear* (1983), described how psychoanalysts intuitively use their own unconscious minds to detect and decipher the unconscious wishes and fantasies of their patients. According to Reik, analysts come to understand patients most deeply by examining their own unconscious intuitions about their patients. Regular meditation practice helps weed out distractions and gives the monkey in our mind repose.

Paul Ekman is a leading researcher in the study of nonverbal communication. In his work (Ekman & Friesen, 1978; Ekman, 2003), Ekman offers an important technical advance in the understanding of nonverbal communication. Before Ekman's research, the emotions passing across our faces were as difficult to analyze as the effect of a gust of wind against a snowbank.

Ekman and his associate Wallace Friesen, both psychologists at the University of California at San Francisco, developed a scientific way to interpret every possible human expression (Ekman, 2003). Their Facial Action Coding System (FACS) has become an essential tool in the science of reading faces. The FACS atlas, available on CD-ROM, describes all 43 movements, or "action units," one's face can perform. In Ekman's class on cultivating emotional balance, students learn to spot expressions projected for anywhere from 1 second to less than one-fifth of a second. Ekman explains that these "microexpressions" can be the most important back channel in a conversation because they are involuntary and reveal what isn't being said with words. In addition, a raised voice pitch, a series of swallows, speech pauses, and repetitions reinforce what the face can tell us.

Attending to nonverbals is not solely the province of counterintelligence agents. Ekman claims that it's a latent ability within all of us; but if we are focusing more on nodding or leaning in while our speaker speaks, we may miss crucial information that could change the course of treatment or signal a patient's hidden agenda.

One important finding is that the upper part of the face expresses feelings almost involuntarily, while we have greater voluntary control over the lower half of our face (Ekman, 2003). When we listen mindfully, we not only pick up more of the telling micro-expressions, but we also note any asymmetries in the tone of voice or the words being said. As practice, try watching a talk show (*Larry King Live* is good for practice as the guests are often fairly close up and facing the camera). Turn down the volume and try to get a sense of how they are feeling about what is being asked. Watch both halves of the face and note split second expressions particularly during pressing questions. Helping patients with nonverbal learning disability or Asperger syndrome identify feelings and moods associated with nonverbal expressions can augment their capacity for interpersonal connection. Ekman's website (*www.paulekman.com*) offers training materials for nonverbal communication well suited for individual and group therapy.

GOING TO THE MOVIES

A helpful way to approach listening deeply is the *movie mind-set*. Even the most dismal listeners will agree that the one place where they listen really well is at the movies. We have all had the experience of becoming engrossed in someone's story. Granted, some stories are more captivating than others, but it is important to remember that patients bring not only their difficulties, but also their own wisdom. The clinician's job is to help them connect to this. We are no help to them if we become attached to their experience, but we be a great help if we can accept and try to understand their experience.

At the movies, however, we are all good listeners. We go to the movies to forget ourselves and our personal soap operas and to explore a different kind of experience. We hunker down with popcorn and a soft drink and get to know the characters we'll be spending the next couple of hours with. As the plot unfolds, we study the motivations and reactions of the main characters attentively. Even if the protagonist is nefarious, our curiosity transcends our judgment of his actions. We feel no need to interrupt, although we may mutter a comment or chuckle. As we become intimate observers of the lives of the characters, we feel their joy or sorrow without losing our perspective that we are in a theater, after all. Close-ups supply us with a wealth of nonverbal information to better understand why this person does the things he does. It is a kind of mindfulness practice; and by the end of the feature we are changed just a bit.

Think back on what movies taught you and how they helped you see life differently. *Old Yeller* softened our hearts for cream-colored labrador retrievers. *Forrest Gump* reminded us that we can learn a lot from simple-minded people. *Scarface* warned us about the dangers in the drug-dealing world. Movies and reality shows fuel that curiosity for seeing life through another lens. Every client you see is a movie for you to experience. Patients and students of mindful listening relate quite well to the movie mind-set. The movie-watching experience is something so familiar that it is easy to apply first in relaxed listening situations and gradually in more challenging listening situations.

Moments when we can share the movie of our own life with an attentive audience are special. All eyes are on us. There are no interruptions. When we pause to think, they listen harder. They never shift their eyes to the clock. We feel a sense of trust. We aren't reprimanded for our point of view. There is unconditional acceptance and respect—the same feeling we want our patients to experience in our presence.

LISTENING AND GENDER

It is so easy to blame others for making it difficult to listen or for not listening to us. One of the most common complaints voiced by couples are the problems of listening. Some of the frustration subsides when couples learn that men and women have different brains, that they process language differently, and that therefore they communicate differently (Pease & Pease, 2000). Drawings of the male and female brains help patients understand these differences. Women's brains have more hot spots for language. Women tend to think aloud and speak a few thousand words more a day than a man. Women also have a thicker corpus callosum (the midline strip that connects the two hemispheres of the brain), allowing for greater integration between left and right hemispheres (Pease & Pease, 2000) of the brain.

Joseph Lurito (2000) of the Indiana University School of Medicine in Indianapolis used functional magnetic resonance imaging to observe 20 men and 20 women while they listened to taped excerpts of John Grisham's novel *The Partner.* In men, listening to these excerpts resulted in increased blood flow to the left temporal lobes. In women, *both* temporal lobes showed increased blood flow. This study suggests why women can handle listening to two conversations at once—because more of their brain is devoted to it. One possibility is that women listen for different things when they hear someone telling a story. The difference in brain activity might reflect a woman's response to the emotional content of the words. Lurito emphasized that "different doesn't mean that one is *better* than another."

A general observation is that men will typically make less eye contact when a woman is speaking, leading women to believe that their male partners are not listening. As Deborah Tannen (1986) pointed out, men prefer a *report* (facts, information) and women like to establish *rapport* in a conversation. Men will not typically pursue a topic at great length like a woman might, and women will ask more questions. Being aware of these physiologically based differences and sharing this knowledge with our patients may help all parties better tolerate and adapt to each gender's communication style.

LISTENING TO OURSELVES

This brings us to the fourth characteristic of a mindful listener—*listening to ourselves.* How well do your words match your intent? Are you aware that the tone of your voice can turn the nicest words sour? What is your ratio of inspiriting (positive, uplifting) to dispiriting (discouraging or patronizing) language? Do you talk too much? Listening to ourselves is probably the greatest challenge in becoming a mindful listener. It requires a sensitivity to our listener's barriers and self-control.

A well-known Zen story teaches us a lot about listening. A university professor wanted to learn about Zen, so he arranged to meet with a Japanese Zen master. The master could see that the professor was already full of knowledge and wanted to impress the master with it. While the master listened patiently to the professor demonstrate his knowledge, he began pouring a cup of tea for the professor. The master filled the cup but kept pouring anyway. At some point the professor noticed the tea spilling across the table and stopped talking. He said, "Master why do you continue to pour the tea? My cup is already full. It can't hold any more." The master replied, "Like this cup you are already full of your own speculations and opinions. How can I teach you Zen unless you first empty your cup?" Clearly there are three interpretations worthy of discussion. One is the obvious: if you start drinking (your *tea*, that is) you'll stop talking. Second, if you start drinking maybe you'll learn something. And third, if you empty your mind (beginner's mind) perhaps you'll have space for new knowledge.

As an exercise I often ask patients to tape themselves during several phone conversations, so they can hear what works and what doesn't. They are often stunned to hear how little they listen in proportion to how often they talk. Rolling their eyes, they'll comment on how difficult it was for them to get to the point or let their conversational partner finish their sentence. Perhaps it was their volume, their tone, the cluttered speech or the repetitive negative or sarcastic undertones that made that conversation fail. In session we start out talking about what went right, then move on to the less effective habits. Then we role play a more effective approach to the conversation.

THE LISTENING STOPPERS

Listening stoppers cause breakdowns in conversations. They include the mis-speaks and behaviors that discourage a listener from wanting to keep the conversation going.

In my ADD support group, listening is one of our favorite topics because we spend much time laughing at the listening mistakes that get us into trouble. Edward Hallowell (Hallowell & Ratey, 2005) describes the ADD brain as "a brain with a Ferrari engine, but with Chevrolet brakes." I set an old statue of laughing Buddha on the table to remind everyone that if we can find humor in our weaknesses, then change does not have to be suffering. Rather it is through greater awareness and acceptance that positive change occurs.

There are several myths about listening that weaken our willingness to improve our skills. Many of us grew up thinking that good listening was an admirable quality associated with a high IQ, granted to a select few. These were the "smart" kids who never had to take a note and had perfect grades. The notion was, if you were not extremely intelligent, you could not hope to become a great listener. Others think that listening is a form of agreeing, or that it is the speaker, not the listener, who is the most powerful one in the conversation.

Another misconception is that good listening takes *more time.* George Wolff, MD, a family physician who has practiced in Greensboro, North Carolina, for more than 40 years and now teaches medicine, claims that if a clinician lets a patient speak for 3 to 4 minutes, he or she will tell the clinician 90% of the diagnosis. Time is something I don't have much of these days; therefore, even with the most verbose of patients and coworkers, I have to set limits in person and on the phone. Many patients know that they go off on tangents and don't mind being brought back on topic. Some are oblivious to the nonverbal cues that signal that their listener's attention has long since wandered. Other times these talkative people are so lost in their own movie that even if I walked out of the room, they would continue talking. This is when a visual cue (e.g., getting out of the chair or raising an index finger) is necessary. Patients generally accept these gentle reminders as long as they feel that the therapist listened mindfully within the session. These cues can also be taught to family members to reduce frustration at home. What really takes up a lot of time (ask a risk management specialist how long a malpractice deposition can take) is *not listening.* Think of the time you have spent mending those communication breakdowns, revising what you *meant* to say, stopping as many as four people on the street for directions, showing up to the meeting on the wrong date at the right time, and so forth. Poor listening wastes time.

Interruption is by far the most annoying listening stopper. It signals disrespect and a lack of patience. Interruptions can be verbal (butting in and changing the subject) or physical (repositioning oneself in a chair, looking at one's watch, etc.). Persons with ADD and anxiety often interrupt the speaker because if they don't, they will forget what they wanted to ask. Interruptions often lead to tangents, or to the listener taking control of the conversation. In such cases, I ask my clients to try to refresh the movie mind-set, take notes, or just breathe while the speaker talks. The questions they don't remember, they admit, were not that important in retrospect. The tendency to interrupt is stronger in social situations where anxiety plays a role. In that case I encourage them to let their conversational partner know that although they may interrupt from time to time, it is not out of disrespect, but as a way of keeping track of information.

In session we often listen to tapes of two-person conversations (parent/teen, husband/wife, manager/employee, etc.). In these dialogues, episodes of interruption are frequent, followed often by advice giving, the next most common listening stopper. When I ask my patients to estimate what percentage of the time during an average interaction advice giving takes place, they estimate it to be about 90% when they are the receiver of the advice. In actuality, when we reviewed the interaction, advice giving took up about a third to a half the time, while rebuttal, stonewalling, cross-complaining, and name calling taking up the rest of the time. The words "should," "never," and "always" echo throughout the discussion.

The irony about advice giving is that it is usually well meaning, straight from the heart. It is a gift we love to give but hate to receive, unless it's requested. Parents share their advice in order to prevent their child from making the same mistakes they did. Parents want to see their children successful and happy, and much to the dismay of their children, the parents are convinced that they know exactly how to make that happen. With couples, the more dominant and protective spouse will feel it his or her responsibility to solve the problem by giving advice. Advice giving only becomes heated and stressful when the receivers of advice shut down and stop listening. A more productive, but active problem-solving discussion involves putting aside our personal agenda and asking our conversational partners first whether *they* have any solutions. Mindful listening keeps the focus on the *process* of sifting through options, thus preserving the relationship. The general rule of thumb is that if they want your advice, they will ask for it. When we start to relinquish control of the conversation, our advice giving subsides. Children and spouses notice the difference almost immediately and the relationship takes a turn for the better. In fact, a son of one of my patients, once the victim of relentless advice, reported after a conversation with his mother that he was genuinely concerned his mother must be on drugs. "She hardly said anything . . . she really *listened* to me . . . it was like we were 'friends' . . . now that's really weird!"

Denying a speaker's reality is another great disconnect. After interruption and advice giving, denial can be a silent and deadly weapon. "You don't mean that" or "It's not that bad, stop exaggerating" or "It's just a turtle, we can get you another one" can be maddening to the child or spouse who's trying to share feelings and experience. The denial of a person's reality can be subtle (trying to cheer up the inconsolable) to extreme (the silent treatment or stonewalling). Denial can be one of the most challenging listening stoppers to change.

A colleague was working with a couple who had reached a communication impasse in their marriage. The exercise during that evening session was to practice accepting each other's feelings without passing judgment. The wife listened patiently to her husband's reasons for his gambling and infidelity and, as the exercise required, reflected his reality appropriately with an understandable degree of reluctance. When it was her turn to share how his behavior had affected her and their children, her husband rolled his eyes and shook his head, adding to his wife's frustration. Unfettered by his wife's heart-wrenching account of his behavior the husband sighed, looked to the therapist and said (referring to himself), "Somebody has to be the sane one!"

As a way to curb the listening stoppers ask yourself four questions: Is what I'm about to say *kind*? Is it *true*? Is it *necessary*, and is it an *improvement upon the silence*? If it passes those tests, I speak. Otherwise, I watch, wait, and listen.

THE LISTENING HELPERS

In this section we discuss the listening helpers, the promoters of positive connection. Allowing attentive, mindful silence is always welcome. Asking "Is there anything else you want to tell me?" or "What are your suggestions?" can steer the interaction in a more constructive direction.

Paraphrasing or telling back in summary form ("Ok, let me see if I heard you right . . . "), used *in moderation*, can keep all parties clear that the intended message was received correctly. This should be used in moderation because some do not appreciate having their thoughts paraphrased. I advise patients to paraphrase if they are being accused of not listening, or if there are many facts to keep in mind as the discussion moves forward. If overused, paraphrasing can become parrotlike and mechanical. Its purpose is to clarify, to assist with a delayed processing problem, or to help one remember what was said. Parents can be encouraged to ask their children to paraphrase directions to help them follow through on tasks. Patients with deficits in auditory processing can learn to paraphrase silently to compensate.

Managing the listening stoppers can be helped by tape review, observation, and role-playing. However, regular mindfulness meditation practice is a first step in taming the listening stoppers. The listening helpers are the manifestation of an accepting and nongrasping mind.

Once a solid core or foundation is set, the mindful communication qualities make sense and more easily become habit, because now it is less work.

CONCLUSION

Today's clinical environment poses challenges to the clinician–patient relationship that would have been unimaginable 50 or more years ago. Despite the hectic schedules, paperwork, and excessive demands on our time, it is possible, through the practice of mindful listening, to shift gears and refocus mental energy on the needs of patients. Being open to receive the *whole* message, sustaining one's attention over time, making patients feel respected, and listening to oneself are the hallmarks of a mindful listener. This kind of listening inspires a sense of partnership, a collaborative and trusting relationship that leads to better outcomes. The hope is that from this therapeutic experience patients will directly or indirectly bring this same quality of communication to their lives outside of the clinic.

At the outset of this chapter I mentioned that I start my day with a prayer. Preparing my mind in this way, internal and external distractions become nothing more than tiny blips in the background; my mind is clear and focused. My long walk down the corridor to meet my next visitor is a meditative one. Let me share it with you:

First, let me consider the mystery of what is about to occur. Let me remember that my patient is a unique being and that my interaction, to the extent that it's genuine, will be unprecedented. Let me remember that each moment is brimming with possibilities, that by listening mindfully, I may be able to heal; by forgoing judgment, I may be able to see more deeply; by letting myself be touched by their experience, I will convey to the patient that I care.

REFERENCES

Benson, H. (1975). *The relaxation response.* New York: William Morrow.

Ekman, P. (2003). *Emotions revealed.* New York: Times Books.

Ekman, P., & Friesen, W. V. (1978). *Facial Action Coding System: A technique for the measurement of facial movements.* Palo Alto, CA: Consulting Psychologists Press.

Glickman, M. (2002). *Beyond the breath: Extraordinary mindfulness through whole body vipassana meditation.* Boston: Journey Editions.

Hallowell, E. M., & Ratey, J. J. (1994). *Driven to distraction*. New York: Simon and Schuster.

Hallowell, E. M., & Ratey, J. J. (2005). *Delivered from distraction*. New York: Ballantine Books.

Lurito, J. T. (2000, November). *Temporal lobe activation demonstrates gender-based differences during passive listening*. Paper presented at the November 2000 meeting of the Radiological Society of North America, Chicago.

Mehrabian, A. (1972). *Nonverbal communication*. Chicago: Aldine-Atherton.

Newberg, A., & D'Aquili, E. (2001). *Why God won't go away*. New York: Ballantine Books.

Nhat Hanh, T. (1987). *The miracle of mindfulness*. Boston: Beacon Press.

Pease, B., & Pease, A. (2000). *Why men don't listen and women can't read maps*. New York: Broadway Books.

Reik, T. (1983). *Listening with the third ear*. New York: Farrar, Straus Giroux.

Shafir, R. Z. (2003). *The Zen of listening: Mindful communication in the age of distraction*. Wheaton, IL: Quest Books.

Tannen, D. (1986). *That's not what I meant: How conversational style makes or breaks relationships*. New York: Ballantine Books.

Epilogue

STEVEN F. HICK
THOMAS BIEN

The benefits to health and well-being from mindfulness and meditation are fairly well established. But mindfulness is more than a technique. And as something more than technique, its full power cannot be captured through mindfulness-based stress reduction (MBSR), mindfulness-based cognitive therapy (MBCT), acceptance and commitment therapy (ACT), or any other specific intervention.

This book has highlighted the potential of mindfulness in fostering an effective therapeutic relationship. The authors agree that the therapeutic relationship is central for effective intervention, and many have concluded that it is more important for client outcome than specialized therapy techniques. Quite likely, this is also true for mindfulness based interventions. Given the centrality of therapeutic relationship and the potential of mindfulness it is surprising that this topic has not received more attention. This book is intended to lay some groundwork in this direction.

As editors we have been privileged to read these innovative accounts of mindfulness and the therapeutic relationship. Within them are several unifying themes that warrant further attention. The authors agree that successful therapists are understanding, accepting, empathic, warm, and supportive. There is broad consensus that decreasing attachment to internal feelings (also discussed as affect regulation) is central for the therapeutic relationship, and agreement that the cultivation of positive attitudes such as caring, kindness, compassion, joy, and equanimity can enhance the therapeutic relationship. Some refer to these attitudes as therapeutic presence. While the terms may be different the intentions are very similar. Deep listening, sometimes expressed through reflection, is perhaps the most commonly cited quality for a mindful therapeutic relationship. Listening as it is described in this volume is much more than hearing the words of the clients or even than attending to nonverbal cues. Mindful listening also involves listening to our biases as they are manifested in our efforts to understand. In the words of Rebecca Shafir, mindful listeners listen to themselves.

There are areas of disagreement, and clearly further research is needed. While some assume that the capacity for a deep, therapeutic relationship correlates with therapist experience, others find that experience can often get in the way. As Russell Walsh put it, "In the moments when therapists believe with certainty that they understand something, they may in fact have lost their way." The relative importance of technique in client outcome may be another area of dispute. Some see the application of their specific therapeutic model as encompassing relationship whereas others see the therapeutic relationship as separable from technique and as a paramount and neglected field. Marlatt, for example, sees the quality of the therapeutic alliance in the treatment of addictive behavior problems as perhaps the most critical factor in determining treatment outcome.

While none of the authors represented in this volume would dispute that the therapeutic relationship is of central, even critical importance, there are clear differences in these writings concerning the extent to which technique is emphasized. Jeremy Safran's work, growing out of the psychoanalytic tradition, emphasizes relational factors more than technique, while authors whose work grows out of the behavioral tradition (Wilson, Marlatt) seem, at least on the surface, to be discussing technique even when thinking about relationship. This is not to suggest the superiority of one emphasis over the other, but to note a difference in emphasis that grows logically from the historical origins of different approaches.

Research to establish that the use of mindfulness by therapists cultivates the qualities necessary for effective therapeutic relationship is just beginning, as Steven Hick notes in Chapter 1. These studies have limitations, but at least serve to illustrate the value of mindfulness for the therapeutic relationship. We believe that further work in this area will be in the vanguard of developments in psychology and related fields.

Stepping back a bit from our normal methodological biases, one can ask, is this drive to objectively prove the value of mindfulness the optimal way to proceed? The field of mindfulness intuitively seems antithetical to objectification and measurement. If mindfulness is truly a way of being that is preconceptual (meaning that one embodies it), then the push to objectify it using abstracted conceptual practices seems paradoxical at best, if not even contradictory. Our scientific research methodologies are squarely based on positivist thinking—with the belief that knowledge can come only from positive affirmation of theories through strict scientific method. Mindfulness seems to approach knowledge and understanding from a more phenomenological perspective—holding that inquiry should focus upon the encountering of objects as lived experience. So the question seems unavoidable: can we use conceptual positivist research methodologies to capture and explicate something that is phenomenological? Some of our authors, such as Michael Lambert, argue cogently that the therapeutic relationship requires empirically based measurement, while authors such as Russell Walsh reach into philosophy rather than science to understand, suggesting that one can never fully assume to understand another person.

We of course would not suggest that science has nothing to offer. Even the Dalai Lama, representing an ancient spiritual tradition, acknowledges that science offers powerful tools for understanding the interconnectedness of all life, and that such understanding provides an essential rationale for ethical behavior and the protection of the environment (see *www.mindandlife.org*). But are the current initiatives to operationalize mindfulness and measure it objectively consistent with the embodied nature of mindfulness? Varela, Thompson, and Rosch (1991, p. 27) have suggested that such research initiatives proceed from an embodied, open-ended reflective mode. "Embodied mode" refers to reflection that brings mind and body together. Open-ended reflection is aware of itself as a form of experience that can be done mindfully. This can cut the habitual chain of thoughts and open up new possibilities. Research in a positivist mode tends to see reflection as just reflection *on* experience, rather than the thing in itself. As Paul Fulton states with regard to examining non-self, the research instrument best suited to this concept may be the idiographic analysis of a single case, that is, one's own experience examined under the microscope of mindful attention.

In sum, future research in this area needs to clarify a number of questions. Can teaching mindfulness improve therapeutic outcome? What is the best way to teach this to therapists? How does the practice of mindfulness affect the process of psychotherapy? Is mindfulness, as practiced by the therapist, more helpful with some therapeutic approaches than with others? Beyond this, however, lie important methodological questions, especially, if mindfulness is inevitably a subjective, presymbolic process, do our established empirical methods provide the best way to study it? Answers to these and many more questions lie ahead.

REFERENCE

Varela, F. J., Thompson, E., & Rosch, E. (1991). *The embodied mind: Cognitive science and human experience.* Cambridge, MA: MIT Press.

Index

Page numbers followed by an *n*, *f*, or *t* indicate notes, figures, or tables.